the healing power of the breath

the healing power
of the breath

Simple Techniques to
Reduce Stress and Anxiety,
Enhance Concentration, and
Balance Your Emotions

Richard P. Brown, MD

Patricia Gerbarg, MD

Shambhala
BOSTON & LONDON
2012

Note to the reader: This book and CD are not intended as substitutes for medical advice or treatment.

Shambhala Publications, Inc.
Horticultural Hall
300 Massachusetts Avenue
Boston, Massachusetts 02115
www.shambhala.com

9 8 7 6 5 4 3

Printed in the United States of America
♾ This edition is printed on acid-free paper that meets the American National Standards Institute z39.48 Standard.
♻ This book is printed on 30% postconsumer recycled paper. For more information please visit www.shambhala.com.
Distributed in the United States by Random House, Inc.,
and in Canada by Random House of Canada Ltd

Interior design and composition by Greta D. Sibley

Library of Congress Cataloging-in-Publication Data

Brown, Richard P.
The healing power of the breath: simple techniques to reduce stress and anxiety, enhance concentration, and balance your emotions / Richard Brown, Patricia Gerbarg.
p.   cm.
ISBN 978-1-59030-902-5 (PBK.)
1. Breathing exercises—Therapeutic use. 2. Mind and body. 3. Health. I. Gerbarg, Patricia L. II. Title.
RA782.B76 2012
613'.192—dc23
2011042585

Contents

the healing power of the breath

Introduction

The Healing Power of Breath

> May suffering ones be suffer-free.
> May the fearstruck fearless be.
> May the grieving shed all grief.
> May all beings find relief.
>
> — *Venerable U Vimalaramsi*

Throughout history, great healers have discovered the power of breathing to enhance the physical, mental, and spiritual well-being of their people. Once secret and sacred, breath practices are now available to everyone. We invite you on a journey through our book and the *Healing Power of the Breath* CD to learn simple, natural methods to become calmer, overcome stress, boost energy, focus your mind, enhance physical fitness, sleep peacefully, and feel closer to those you love. We will teach you core breathing techniques, explain how they work, and show you how to use them to meet the many challenges you face.

The human body has the power to heal itself from the cellular level up. We regenerate our body tissues every day. Before the advent of synthetic medications, shamans, monks, priests, and tribal leaders learned how to turn on the body's natural abilities to prevent and cure illness. Breathing practice (*pranayama*) is one of the classical limbs of yoga and can be found in modern yoga studios all around the world. While yoga practitioners and martial artists employ breath techniques, the modern science of breath is exploring the vast healing potential of the human respiratory system.

Studies are revealing that by changing the patterns of breathing it is possible to restore balance to stress response systems, calm an agitated mind, relieve symptoms of anxiety and post-traumatic stress disorder (PTSD), improve physical health and endurance, elevate performance, and enhance relationships. The scientific bases for such powerful effects of breathing practices will be presented as we show how to use them in many aspects of your daily life.

What do Mahatma Gandhi, the martial artist Bruce Lee, Buddhist meditators, Christian monks, Hawaiian *kahuna*s, and Russian Special Forces have in common? They all used breathing to enhance their physical, mental, and spiritual well-being. For instance, Mahatma Gandhi, who embodied the principles of righteous action and nonviolence, enjoyed chanting his prayers every morning. The demands he faced in leading the people of India by peaceful resistance through their struggle for independence from the British were certainly on a larger scale than most of our own day-to-day stresses. Just as chanting helped Gandhi guide his people through dangerous times, it can help keep your stress-response systems in balance through whatever challenges you face. When the famous martial artist and actor Bruce Lee bellowed before delivering a lethal blow, he was not just making noise to terrify his opponent. The great breath behind the shout sharpened his senses and primed his body for the strike. A practice we call Breath Moving was highly developed by medieval Russian Orthodox Christian monks who used it prior to reciting the Jesus Prayer and to attain higher spiritual states. These monks shared their breath secrets to fortify the holy Christian knights who were defending Russia from waves of invaders, and traces of their practices can be found in the training of today's Russian Special Forces. Knowledge of breath practices was also passed down through generations of great kahunas in the mountains of

Hawaii; Hawaiian breath techniques of the present day are similar in many ways to those found in India and China.

The presence of related ancient breath forms in so many different areas of the world suggests that their roots must go back in time, perhaps ten thousand years or more. For example, slow breathing at rates of five to six breaths per minute are found in yoga, qigong, and Buddhist meditation.

This book will introduce you to knowledge and modern research on stress reduction through breathwork that is just as relevant to health in modern life as it was in ancient times. The stresses of modern life induce negative emotions such as anxiety, frustration, anger, and cynicism. In addition, stress accelerates the decline in physical health due to cardiovascular disease, obesity, inflammation, and immune dysfunction. The daily use of breath practices can turn back the tide of stress, counteract disease progression, and improve overall quality of life. Along with its physical toll, stress is also wearing on the spirit: it can lead to the buildup of emotional defenses that choke off our capacity for love, compassion, and intimacy. Breath practices combined with self-reflection can unlock the metal casing around the heart, enabling reconnection with loving feelings and positive emotions within ourselves and in our relationships.

How to Use This Book and the Accompanying CD

Much of this book is to be used in tandem with the accompanying *Healing Power of the Breath* CD to teach a series of core breath practices and supplementary techniques. Chapters 1, 2, and 3 will teach you a sequence of core practices: Coherent Breathing, Resistance Breathing, Breath Moving, the Total Breath, and Body Scan. Be sure to start at the beginning and work your way through the chapters, because each one builds upon the others. First read through the instructions on how to do each breath practice. Then find the matching track on the CD. Let the CD pace your breathing and guide your practice. Take time to ensure that you can do each technique smoothly and comfortably without straining before you move on to the next chapter. For example, you may choose to practice the technique we call Coherent Breathing for ten minutes once or twice a day for a few days before trying Resistance Breathing. After that, take a few days to work on Coherent and Resistance Breathing before starting Breath Moving.

In the beginning, when practicing breath techniques, it is best to give them your full attention and minimize distractions. Find a quiet spot. Ask your friends and family not to interrupt you. Turn off your cell phone or PDA. Sit in a very comfortable chair or lie down.

There are hundreds of different breathing practices, each with its own merits. In this book, we have chosen to focus on just a few that we find to be the most useful, rapidly effective, and easy to learn. Another criterion we use is safety. Having taught thousands of people breathing practices, we have learned that some people are vulnerable to adverse reactions. Therefore, we offer only practices that are safe for everyone. We call the first four the core practices, but in fact some of them are quite advanced. For example, in traditional yoga training, one might have to study for years before being allowed to learn some of these techniques.

In ancient times, yoga students were expected to practice many hours daily—and for many years. The goals of yoga were extensive and lofty: the union of mind, body, and spirit, and ultimately spiritual enlightenment. Advanced practices were reserved for only the most devoted students. While there are serious yoga students today who devote many years to their studies, the majority of people, particularly in Western cultures, do not choose to pursue yoga as an intense spiritual or religious discipline. Most Westerners are interested in yoga as a physical exercise or as a method to relax. These more circumscribed goals can be achieved more rapidly with a modest investment of time by using specific breath practices. We focus on gentle breath practices that can be learned by novices as well as experienced yoga students. The pursuit of more intense breath practices would require more time and preparation with a teacher.

Once you master the first three core practices, you will be able to perform what we call the Total Breath, a gentle, powerful, versatile practice that can be used to alleviate many aspects of mental and physical suffering.

If you have only twenty minutes for yourself in the course of your day, we recommend you use it for the Total Breath. In addition, in chapters 4 and 5, you will discover more techniques including "Ha" Breath, Breath Counts, and Vibration Breathing.

Chapters 5, 6, and 7 explain the many ways to use the techniques learned in earlier chapters to manage stress, insomnia, anxiety, depression, post-traumatic stress, difficulties in relationships, physical pain, artistic expression, and athletic performance. The effects of breath practices on the brain, emotion regulation, stress-response systems, hormones, negative and positive emotions, and the capacity to feel love will be discussed, including some of the supporting scientific evidence. We will share stories about our students, our patients, and ourselves to illustrate some of the ways that breath practices can make a difference in people's lives. Certain details have been changed in the case histories in order to protect the privacy of our patients who have generously offered to share their stories. Many of the questions that arise when people are learning to use these techniques will be addressed in each chapter. If you cannot find an answer within the chapters, you are welcome to write to us at www.haveahealthy mind.com and we will do our best to answer your questions about the practices. Tables in the appendix provide a quick summary of when and how to use each of the practices taught in this book. The final pages of the book also offer a list of resources where you can find instructors, workshops, CDs, DVDs, books, and other information to pursue your interests in mind-body approaches to health and wellness.

Asthma, Obstructive Lung Disease, Reactive Airway Disease

If you have asthma, chronic obstructive pulmonary disease (COPD), reactive airway disease, toxic inhalant exposure, or another serious medical condition, take time to read the section on asthma in chapter 3 before you begin the breath practices. We also suggest that you check with your doctor to be sure that it is safe for you to do breath practices. In the long run, breathing exercises will improve most respiratory conditions. However, in the beginning, it is often necessary to modify the practices. Chapter 1 will tell you how to do the necessary modifications so that you can use "the breathing cure" safely.

The Breath Practice CD

Inside the back cover of this book you will find the *Healing Power of the Breath* CD. The chapters in this book explain how to use the CD to guide the breath practices. The CD has the following tracks:

Track 1   Introduction

Track 2   Instruction: Coherent Breathing Chime Track at 5 bpm
(5 minutes)

Track 3   Instruction: Resistance Breathing (3 minutes)

Track 4   Instruction: Breath Moving with Coherent Breathing
(6 minutes)

Track 5   Instruction and Practice: "Ha" Breath (2 minutes)

Track 6   Instruction and Practice: Breath Counts 4-4-6-2 (2 minutes)

Track 7   Instruction and Practice: Om and Song Kong Tong Dong
(5 minutes)

Track 8   Practice: Total Breath with Chime Track at 5 bpm
(21 minutes)

Track 9   Practice: Body Scan (5 minutes)

Track 10   Practice: Total Breath with Chime Track at 6 bpm
(21 minutes)

Track 11   Practice: Body Scan (5 minutes)

Additional Recommended Aids for Breath Practice

Stephen Elliot has created additional aids for learning coherent breathing. For those who would like more variety in sound tracks, who need additional rhythms, or who are hearing impaired, visit his Web site, www.coherence.com.

1. *Slow Down!* is a CD recommended for people who find it difficult to slow their breathing down to five breaths per minute as quickly as instructed in our book. People who have lung diseases or restricted breathing may need to take more time. Also, some people with extremely high levels of anxiety may need more time to adjust their breathing. If you find that you are not able to slow your breathing down to five or six breaths per minute as you work through chapter 1, after trying for several days, then it may be better for you to start with the *Slow Down!* CD available on the Web site www.coherence.com. This will ease you in more gradually. *Slow Down!* allows you to start with your natural rate and then gradually reduce it using rhythms that range from nineteen to five breaths per minute. See chapter 1 for further instructions.

2. The Coherence Clock is an audiovisual computer application that serves as a "breathing pacemaker." The clock that appears on the screen has a second hand that moves from twelve to six for exhalation and from six to twelve for inhalation. A "tick" occurs with each advance of the hand. The application enables people with hearing impairment to follow the visual cues of the clock rather than sounds. You can find the Coherence Clock at www.coherence.com.

3. Another audio resource for pacing in breath practices is offered by Stephen Elliot at the Web site www.coherence.com. For those who would like more variety in sound tracks, who need additional rhythms, or who are hearing impaired, his *Respire-1* CD includes an instructional track, Tibetan bell tracks, and a voice-paced track. Most people enjoy the chime sounds, but some people, including those who have suffered from concussions or other brain injuries, do not tolerate the chime vibrations well. In this case, the voice track is useful and recommended.

Healing breath techniques are for everyone. They will not take you long to learn. In fact many people are able to learn the first breath form, Coherent Breathing, in just thirty minutes or less. However, if it takes you longer, just be patient and you will see that it becomes easier and easier as you practice. While breath practices have the power to heal, they require your active participation in order to be effective. Some people find it easier to quickly take a pill than to set aside twenty minutes of time to practice breathing every day. However, if you prefer to activate the natural healing processes within your body, to reconnect with your true self, and to experience more meaningful relationships—treasures not found in a pill bottle—then this book is for you. With a little time and effort you will soon be able to harness the power of the breath to enhance your health and happiness.

I

The Sweetest Spot

Coherent Breathing and the Body Scan

Can you focus your life-breath until you become supple as a newborn child?

—*Lao Tzu*, Tao Te Ching

Babies are remarkably flexible. They can put a toe in their mouth almost as easily as a thumb. Not only their joints, but many other parts of their bodies are more elastic than those of adults. As we age, we become less elastic, more rigid, both physically and mentally. The walls of the blood vessels of a baby are far more elastic than those of an adult who may develop "hardening of the arteries" in old age. The responsiveness of a baby's nervous system is also more flexible. It is this flexibility that enables infants and children to respond and adapt more rapidly to a greater range of environmental changes. When a person is highly adaptable, their system undergoes less wear and tear during the challenges and stresses of everyday life. Stress resilience is the capacity to recover and rebound from challenging events. Everyone has the capacity to increase their stress resilience. We just need to turn up the healing, recharging parts of the nervous system and tone down the overreactive part of the system. Breath practices enable us to fine-tune the stress response systems quickly whenever needed.

When an individual experiences more stress than their system can handle, particularly repeated or prolonged stress, there will be adverse effects on their emotional and physical health. Initially the person may just feel some tension, excess worry, and some difficulty falling asleep. This can progress to actual anxiety, obsessive worry, insomnia, daytime fatigue, irritability, and muscle aches. During this time, the stress-response system is doing its best to cope, possibly by releasing more cortisol, more adrenaline, more excitatory neurotransmitters, all of which burns more energy, releases more free radicals, and increases inflammation. However, if this goes on too long, the stress-response system may become exhausted, leading to a state of depression, chronic fatigue, overreactivity, feelings of being overwhelmed or helpless, and the progression of physical illnesses such as cardiovascular disease. It is possible to prevent or even reverse this progression by increasing the strength, balance, and resilience of the stress response system.

Coherent Breathing and Heart Rate Variability

In order to cultivate stress resilience, we begin with belly breathing and Coherent Breathing, techniques that shift the stress-response system into a healthier balance by activating the healing, recharging part of the nervous system while quieting the defensive, energy-burning parts. After you learn Coherent Breathing, we will teach you a relaxation practice that will also produce a noticeable increase in the flexibility of your cardiovascular system. The healing effects of Coherent Breathing are accelerated by the addition of techniques such as Resistance Breathing and Breath Moving. Most people are just too busy to spend hours on mind-body practices. We have combined three breath practices into one technique, which we call Total Breath, to maximize the impact and minimize the length of practice time.

The healing, calming part of the nervous system is the parasympathetic nervous system. The level of activity of this system can be measured using the natural fluctuations in heart rate that are linked to breathing; these fluctuations are used to calculate heart rate variability, or HRV. Changing the rate and pattern of breathing alters HRV, reflecting shifts in nervous system activity. We know this not only from scientific studies but also from trying it ourselves and observing its effects in our patients and students. You can do a simple test of this on yourself. Sit comfortably and place two fingers on your pulse, either on the side of your neck or on your wrist, whichever is easier. Now breathe slowly and deeply. Continue the slow deep breathing as you count your pulse. Count the number of beats when you breathe in, and compare it with the number of beats when you breathe out. What do you notice? If you found that your heart beats faster when you breathe in than when you breathe out, you are correct. You have discovered that every breath you take affects your heart rate. Heart rate variability not only responds to breathing in and breathing out, it also changes with the overall rate of breathing. For example, breathing slowly increases HRV. Is that good? Since changes in HRV are mediated through the autonomic nervous system, when the HRV is higher it means that the system adjusting the heart rate as you breathe in and out is responding more robustly and more flexibly to changes in breathing. When HRV is low, it means that either something is impaired or the system is aging and becoming more rigid. So the answer is yes, increasing HRV is very good, because having a higher HRV is associated with a healthier, more flexible cardiovascular system, a more balanced and resilient stress-response system, and overall greater health and longevity. In fact, scientists use HRV as a means of measuring the balance of the stress-response system and a balanced stress response means less wear and tear on the body. People with anxiety disorders, depression, post-traumatic stress, attention deficit disorder, excess aggression, cardiovascular disease, and irritable bowel syndrome have reduced HRV and dysfunctions in their stress response systems.[1] After you learn Coherent Breathing, we will teach you a relaxation practice that will also demonstrate the increased flexibility of your cardiovascular system.

Coherent Breathing is a simple way to increase heart-rate variability and balance the stress-response systems. When scientists tested people at all possible breathing rates, they found that there is an ideal breath rate for each person, somewhere between three and a half and six breaths per minute for adults using equal time for breathing in and breathing out, a sweet spot where the HRV is maximized and the electrical rhythms of the heart, lungs, and brain become synchronized. Modern researchers have called this the resonant rate,[2] but this phenomenon has been known for centuries by religious adepts in many cultures. For example, when Zen Buddhist monks enter deep meditation, called *zazen,* they breathe at six breaths per minute.[3] The Italian cardiologist Luciano Bernardi discovered that traditional chanting of the Latin Hail Mary occurs at six breaths per minute.[4] In chapter 7 you will learn more about Bernardi's fascinating studies, in which resonant breathing enhanced high-altitude performance.

Coherent Breathing is breathing at a rate of five breaths per minute, around the middle of the resonant breathing rate range. Tracks 8 and 10 on the *Healing Power of the Breath* CD that accompanies this book will pace your breathing with a chime tone at five and six breaths per minute, respectively. We use these rates because they maximize HRV for most people. Breathing at a rate that is close to one's ideal resonant rate can induce up to a tenfold improvement in HRV.[5] For people who are over six feet tall, the ideal resonant rate is three to three and a half breaths per minute. For children under the age of ten, comfortable rates range between six and ten breaths per minute. Although most adolescents and adults can learn to breathe at five breaths per minute easily, some people have more difficulty due to physical issues such as asthma or obstructive lung disease. High levels of body tension can also impede attempts to slow down the breath. To make it easier for those who need more time to adjust to slow breathing, *The Healing Power of the Breath* CD provides track 10 to pace breathing at six breaths per minute.

There are many ways to learn Coherent Breathing, including a growing array of commercial gadgets with visual cues. But we prefer a method that is relaxing and easy to use anytime, anywhere. Research shows that keeping the eyes closed and the hands still has significant effects on brain waves, indicating greater relaxing effects. When people look at a computer screen, move their eyes, or type on a keyboard, this activity can interfere with the attainment of optimal states of relaxation. This is one of the reasons why we use breathing. It can be done with eyes closed and hands at rest.

In learning breath practices the most important thing to remember is to relax. That may sound obvious, but it isn't. As you are learning a new practice it may feel awkward or unnatural at first. You may begin to worry about whether you are doing it correctly, whether it is working, whether you need to try harder. All this thinking and worrying will just make you tense up. Self-judgment adds another layer of stress. The less you judge yourself, the easier it will be to relax and experience the benefits of Coherent Breathing. As you read this book, simply follow the instructions as best you can, give yourself time to get the hang of it, and sooner than you imagine, it will all go smoothly. Try not to evaluate or judge what is happening. Just go with it.

Breath Awareness, or Mindfulness of Breath

In the Anapanasati Sutra, an ancient Buddhist text, Buddha taught that awareness of breath was the beginning and the end of the road to enlightenment. The best way to become aware of your breath is to sit comfortably, close your mouth, and breathe through your nose. If you cannot breathe through your nose, you can still do all of the practices by breathing through your mouth with your lips slightly parted. Close your eyes if you are comfortable doing so. Feel the air as it moves in and out of your nose. Breathe slowly and deeply. Feel the air move down into your lungs, then back up and out again. Feel the rise and fall of your belly and chest, the movement of your ribs. Now you are becoming aware of your breath.

Belly Breathing

This part will be easier if you lie down. Make sure your neck and back are comfortable. Use whatever pillows or cushions you may need. Close your eyes, close your mouth, and breathe through your nose. Taking a deep breath in, relax your belly muscles so that your belly rises each time you breathe in. It is not necessary to actively push your belly out. Let the breath fill you, causing your belly to rise naturally, like a balloon filling with air. Then let your belly come down naturally as you breathe out. Repeat this slowly several times. All breathing should be slow and gentle without any straining. Take these deep belly breaths in and out several times as you relax the muscles of your face and let your whole body relax.

If you are not sure which way your belly is moving, place a small object on your navel and watch it move up and down as you breathe. You could use a shoe, a tissue box, or a favorite stuffed animal. When you are comfortable belly breathing with your eyes closed, move on to Coherent Breathing.

Coherent Breathing

You may sit or lie down in a comfortable, supported position. Close your eyes, close your mouth, and breathe through your nose. Focus your attention on feeling the breath move in and out through your nose and airways to your lungs. When other thoughts enter your mind, just let them float through and refocus your attention on the breathing sensations. Breathing should be slow, gentle, comfortable, not forced in any way.

When you are first learning to do Coherent Breathing at five breaths per minute (bpm), you will need to begin in steps to slow down your breath rate. Once you have learned to breathe at five breaths per minute, you will not need to use these starting steps. You will be able to just start the *Healing Power of the Breath* CD and within a few breaths you will be in the correct rhythm. But the first few times, follow the beginning steps listed below.

If you find that trying to breathe at five bpm is too difficult, then as an alternative begin with six bpm using the last track on the CD that accompanies this book. Once you have mastered breathing at six bpm, it will be easier for you to slow down to five bpm, or you may choose to stay with the faster rate.

If you are not able to slow down to six bpm, you may need to begin with Steve Elliot's *Slow Down!* CD. (See the sidebar in the introduction.) This CD begins at your natural breath rate and very gradually slows your breathing down.

Beginning Steps for Coherent Breathing

- Breathe through your nose with your eyes closed.
- Taking your time, count slowly and silently in your mind: As you breathe in, . . . *two* . . . As you breathe out . . . *two* . . . Repeat this for two breaths.
- Taking your time, count slowly: As you breathe in . . . *two* . . . *three* . . . As you breathe out, . . . *two* . . . *three* . . . Repeat this for three breaths.
- Taking your time, count slowly: As you breathe in . . . *two* . . . *three* . . . *four* . . . As you breathe out . . . *two* . . . *three* . . . *four* . . . Repeat this for four breaths.
- Taking your time, count a little more slowly: As you breathe in . . . *two* . . . *three* . . . *four* . . . As you breathe out . . . *two* . . . *three* . . . *four* . . . Repeat this for four breaths.

Once you learn to breathe at five breaths per minute, you will not need to use these learning steps. You will be able to just start the *Healing Power of the Breath* CD and within a few breaths you will be in the correct rhythm.

Play track 2 of the CD. Continue breathing slowly as you listen first to Dr. Brown's voice, and then to the two-bells chime. When you hear one chime tone, breathe in very slowly. When you hear the next chime tone, breathe out very slowly. If you find it difficult to sustain your breath from one tone to the next, it may be because you are breathing too forcefully, inhaling or exhaling the air too quickly. Try to move the air more slowly in and out. This will slow down your breathing and allow you to retain enough air to make it to the next tone. The more slowly and gently you breathe, the easier it will be.

Old tensions are stored in our systems. Feel where the tension is in your body. You may feel the tension in your belly, chest, throat, or neck. Let it go more and more with each out-breath. Imagine the breath as the wind moving through a forest of trees.

Continue the Coherent Breathing practice for five minutes. If it is going smoothly and easily, continue for ten minutes. However, if you are struggling, stop and rest. Relax a bit and then try again. Be patient and give yourself time to adjust to the breathing without judgment. If you are still having difficulties, read "How to Deal with Obstacles to Coherent Breathing," below.

Most people enjoy the gentle sound of the chimes on the *Healing Power of the Breath* CD. However, some people find the human voice to be more soothing. If you prefer to pace your breath using a voice recording, we recommend that you use the *Respire-1* CD recorded by Stephen Elliot. It is available on his Web site, www.coherence.com. On the third track, voice commands are used to pace the breathing. People who have had head trauma often find the voice-led track to be more comfortable and calming. Another reason to use the *Respire-1* CD is that the longer-running tracks are convenient for practicing twenty minutes. The Coherence Web site also allows for direct downloading onto iPods or MP3 players.

Daily Practice of Coherent Breathing

Start with five to ten minutes of Coherent Breathing once or twice a day, either lying down or sitting in a very comfortable chair, and gradually increase up to twenty minutes at a time. Most people notice benefits immediately. You will notice that your mind feels calmer, less filled with chatter; your body feels more relaxed. In the beginning, these good feelings may last only a short time after you get up and start doing things under the usual pressures. However, with practice over time, the benefits will last longer and longer, the sense of calm alertness will grow, and the feelings of tension will fade. You will get some benefits even if you practice irregularly, but if you practice nearly every day, your progress will be much faster and stronger. Once you master Coherent Breathing, you can go right into it without having to slow your breath by counting to four in steps, as we described above for beginners.

There are many ways to use Coherent Breathing:

1. Coherent Breathing for anxiety and trouble sleeping
    Whenever you feel stressed or anxious, use Coherent Breathing. You will find that even five minutes can help you to stop worrying and relax. If you have difficulty falling asleep, just get into bed, turn on the chime track, turn out the light, and breathe yourself to sleep.

2. Coherent Breathing during daily activity
    After three months of regular practice with your eyes closed, you may also begin to do Coherent Breathing with your eyes open. Just play the chime recording and breathe along as you putter around the house, commute on the train, or take a walk. Coherent Breathing is fine for walking, but if you are jogging or exercising, you will need to breathe at a faster rate. Eventually, you will learn how to maintain the Coherent Breathing rate on your own without the chime track. You can even breathe coherently while working on the computer, doing paperwork, taking tests, or any other anxiety-provoking activity. You can download the chime track onto an iPod or MP3 Player and take it wherever you go — for instance, if you are a commuter on the subway you can use it to relax and get ready

for your day. You can even use Coherent Breathing at work. No one will know how slowly you breathe or how you manage to stay so calm when everyone else is freaking out. Eventually, you will be able to shift into Coherent Breathing even without the chime track. At that point, we suggest that you go in and out of Coherent Breathing all day long. It is very healthy and will help to further strengthen and balance your system.

Even after you have mastered Coherent Breathing, it is very beneficial to continue to do it in a focused way for the most powerful effects—try to do it with your eyes closed, using the *Healing Power of the Breath* CD, for about twenty minutes once a day. If you have an anxiety disorder or depression, you will need to practice twenty minutes twice a day, as we will explain in chapter 4.

Your Anchor

Like ships at sea, we are pulled in different directions by the winds of our aspirations and the currents of our desires. The mind pursues excitement, stimulation, challenge, achievement, new ideas, and change. The body prefers comfort, pleasure, and the predictability of regular eating and sleeping schedules. What does the heart desire? Love, tenderness, intimacy, and security. How often do the mind, the body, and the heart all want the very same thing? Not often enough. Moreover, we are constantly subject to demands from the external environment, the needs of others. How do we keep our balance amidst so many demands and desires? One way is to use Coherent Breathing as your anchor. It will induce resonance between your heart and your brain rhythms. Know when you are away from it and return yourself to it. You will find it easier to unify your mind, body, and heart. Visit it every day to be in touch with your original self in both action and stillness—bringing mind, body, and spirit into alignment.

How to Deal with Obstacles to Coherent Breathing

Any time you try something new there may be a glitch. Here are some of the obstacles you may encounter and what to do about them.

Catching Your Breath

What if you find that your breath catches in the middle of the inhale? The catch in the breath probably comes from stress and tension. Don't worry about it. Just continue the breathing practice. You will experience the benefits of Coherent Breathing with or without a catch in your breath. Eventually, when more of the tension has been released through the mind-body practices, you will be able to let go and inhale smoothly. Until then, practice the breathing without dwelling on this catch in your breath. When you are not thinking about it, it will vanish on its own.

Running Out of Breath

Suppose you have tried and tried, but you cannot breathe slowly enough to stay with the chimes. You seem to run out of breath. In the beginning, you may find that you come to the end of your inhale before the next chime. When this occurs, just let your breath pause as you wait for the chime, and then exhale slowly. With time and practice, you will learn to breathe more slowly and gently so that each breath will elongate to reach the chime tone. Remind yourself to breathe more gently and to move the air in and out more and more slowly.

Some people have enough breath to last through the exhale, but not enough to last through the inhale. Most people find it easier to prolong the exhale compared with the inhale, especially in the beginning. Novices tend to draw the air in too quickly. This usually corrects itself over time as you learn to inhale more gently, moving the air more slowly. Some people want to give and give, but have difficulty receiving. As you slow down the inhale, you will be allowing yourself to open up to receive all that the breath has to give you.

If Five Breaths per Minute Feels Too Fast

Some people feel that breathing at five breaths per minute is too fast, and they want to breathe more slowly. Individuals who are well-trained athletes, such as runners or swimmers, may feel this way. Yoga practitioners sometimes want to slow their breathing to four, three, or even two breaths per minute, as they have done during deep meditation.

If you prefer slower rates, that is fine while doing other practices such as deep meditation. However, it is important to learn Coherent Breathing at five breaths per minute and to stay with this rate for the practices we are teaching.

Why not slow down? Isn't slower better? Not necessarily. It depends on your intention. If your goal is to achieve a deeply relaxed meditative state, perhaps one in which you may even let go of conscious awareness, then slower breathing may be appropriate. However, in that kind of state, you would not be able to work or perform tasks requiring attention. Also, slower rates lead to parasympathetic dominance rather than an optimal balance between the parasympathetic and the sympathetic systems.

The unique benefits of Coherent Breathing are attributable to the use of specific rates that induce a state of mental calm coupled with alert awareness, the ideal state for most activities at home, at work, or at play. We find that five breaths per minute is somewhat more calming compared to six breaths per minute, which maximally opens the capillaries to optimize blood flow and oxygenation of the extremities. When your goal is to improve physical performance, especially under conditions of low oxygen (such as high-altitude activities), six breaths per minute would be excellent preparation. Even if five breaths per minute feels too slow for you, unless you are over six feet tall, let the bell tones pace you for Coherent Breathing at five breaths per minute and follow the practices we describe. (As we noted earlier, if you are over six feet tall, your ideal resonant rate is in fact slower: three to three and a half breaths per minute.) In this way, you will discover the special benefits of Coherent Breathing for yourself.

Practicing When Your Nose Is Stuffed Up

If your nose is stuffed up, how can you do the Coherent Breathing? You may breathe through partly closed lips on both the inhale and the exhale until your nasal passages are clear. Breathing through an open mouth can make it a little more difficult to slow down your breath rate, and your throat may become dry and uncomfortable. If a stuffed-up nose is a frequent problem for you, as it often is with allergy sufferers, then you may use pursed lips while doing Coherent Breathing. In chapter 2 we will explain how to breathe correctly with pursed lips. You will be able to use pursed lips effectively on both the in-breath and the out-breath.

You can try some natural methods to clear your nasal passages. For example, tighten your hands into two fists. Press the right fist firmly into the left armpit and the left fist firmly into the right armpit for two minutes. By stimulating sensory nerves, pressure in the left armpit should clear the right nostril while pressure in the right armpit should clear the left nostril. Alternatively, you may need to use mentholated cough drops, an inhaler, a nasal spray, or some form of nasal irrigation, for instance with a neti pot.

Pesky Pets

How can you practice when your pets want attention? What to do with cats and dogs while you practice breathing depends on your pet's temperament. For instance, if your dog tends to pester you, bark, nudge you for attention, or jump on you to play, it may be necessary for you to put your pet out of the room, as this behavior is too distracting. However, if you have a mellow dog who will lie still beside you, your dog can learn to wait quietly for hugs and praise at the end of your practice. Animals respond to human physical cues, including breathing. As you become more and more relaxed, your pets will also tend to become calmer.

Family Needs

No one wants to feel torn between doing their self-healing practices and attending to their family's needs. Very young children may not be able to control their need to be close to you. For instance, one mother told us that her young children would lie close to her quietly during Coherent Breathing, and she believed that by feeling and hearing her breathe, they became calmer, too. Although parents are usually told to practice yoga in isolation, if you have children who don't squirm too much you may be able to focus on your breath practices even with your children nearby. Otherwise, you may need to practice during their naptime or when someone else is available to occupy them.

Clear communication is one of the best ways to avoid negative interactions with your children when you want to do your practices. Enlist the support of your family by explaining that you need to do breathing practices every day in order to reduce stress and improve your energy, mood, and ability to handle your responsibilities, including everything you do for them. Help your family understand that this is your special time and that you are not to be disturbed. Assist them in planning activities to occupy their time while you are practicing. Your children will be the first to sense that you are calmer, less irritable, more patient, and more responsive to them. Once they see the connection between having a calmer, happier, gentler parent and the breathing practice, they will become your most ardent supporters. They may even ask you to teach them some of the techniques. Dr. Gerbarg's teenage son once teased her about the breathing practices, saying, "Mom, you are so chill now. I bet I could ask you for a Porsche and you would say yes." Children can find ways to help parents do their practices, as the following illustrates.

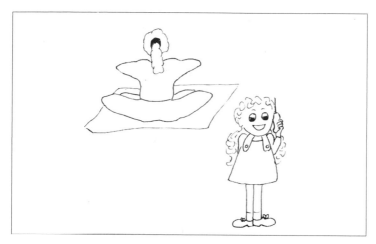

"My mommy can't come to the phone until she stops breathing."

Finding a Time to Breathe

Sometimes it isn't easy to find time to breath during a busy day. When is the best time of day to do breathing practices? Any time you can do the breathing practice is good—morning practice refreshes and calms; evening practice recharges and relaxes for sleep. For instance, one of our patients, Alison, complained of feeling tired all day, stressed out at work, and "crabby" when she got home at night. She was making more mistakes at work and worried about losing her job. We taught her Coherent Breathing during an office appointment, and she was able to experience the relaxing and refreshing effects.

Even though Alison realized that the breath practices worked, she did not want to get up twenty minutes earlier to make time for morning breath practice. She compromised, agreeing to practice for ten minutes in the morning and another ten minutes at the end of the day for one week. She discovered that the morning practice refreshed her and prevented fatigue better than the ten minutes of sleep she had given up. Also, since she was more relaxed throughout the day, she was able to get more work done with better attention to details, fewer mistakes, and smoother interactions with coworkers. Instead of leaving work feeling defeated at the end of the day, she found herself coming home feeling good about what she had accomplished and ready to enjoy her family. Alison's family meant a great deal to her. By the end of the first month she chose to make the breathing practice part of her permanent morning routine and miraculously she found twenty minutes in which to do it.

Sleeping When You Want to Stay Awake

You may become so relaxed that you fall asleep during the breathing practices, even when you want to stay awake. This probably means that you are not getting enough sleep at night. When you don't have to rush off to work and you have the time, it is best to allow yourself this extra rest. Your system may need it. However, when you don't have the time to sleep, you may need to do the breath practices sitting up and using Breath Moving (see chapter 3) to stay awake.

We have seen people with severe sleep deprivation fall asleep during Coherent Breathing, even while sitting up, and sometimes even snoring loudly. If this occurs repeatedly it may be a sign of obstructive sleep apnea (OSA), a condition that requires medical evaluation. Obstructive sleep apnea can be a cause of fatigue, falling asleep while driving, obesity, and pulmonary hypertension.

Feeling Unsafe

Among the hundreds of people who attend our workshops, there are usually some who are survivors of severe abuse or trauma. A person who grows up in an unsafe, abusive environment can have much in common with a war veteran returning from multiple tours of duty—*they never feel safe*. One of the symptoms of post-traumatic stress disorder is hypervigi-lance, meaning a state of always watching out for danger. As a result, the traumatized person may be unable to close his or her eyes when other people are around.

Usually one of us leads our Breath~Body~Mind workshops while the other walks quietly around the room assisting participants who need help with the practices. During one morning workshop, we noticed Bianca, a slim, dark-haired woman sitting bolt upright with her eyes wide open. Dr. Gerbarg asked if she would feel comfortable closing her eyes while learn-ing breath practices. She shook her head no. Bianca never closed her eyes when there were people around. Having grown up in an abusive home, Bianca never felt safe. She suffered from hypervigilance, and she constantly scanned her surroundings for possible threats. Rather than pressure Bianca to close her eyes, Dr. Gerbarg gently suggested that she try to half-close her eyes so that she could focus her attention inward and notice her more sub-tle experiences. Six months later, Bianca returned to take another work-shop. She reported that she had learned to use Coherent Breathing with Resistance Breathing to calm herself whenever feelings of panic arose. Another sign of progress was that during her second workshop she was able to breathe with her eyes completely closed.

The More the Merrier: The Family That Breathes Together . . .

Candace, a mother of two girls, had an eleven-year-old daughter who wanted to do the breathing with her. We advised her that children over the age of ten can usually learn breath practice with a parent, but in the beginning they should only do it for a few minutes or for as long as their natural attention span allows. It is not helpful to insist that a child sit still and do breath practices for longer periods of time. Frustration and restless-ness will defeat the purpose of the practice. If a child maintains an interest, they can do it for longer periods of time, but this should be determined by how they feel.

"What about my six-year-old daughter?" Candace asked. We explained that a younger child needs a faster breath rate than an adult. For children between the ages of five and ten, the simplest method of breath practice is to have them breathe at a rate of ten breaths per minute. For this rate, they do one entire breath, breathing in and breathing out, after each bell tone. In other words, at the sound of each chime they inhale and exhale before the next bell. This paces the child's breathing rhythm to ten breaths per minute while the parent is doing five breaths per minute. A younger child should only do this for a few minutes or for as long as her natural attention span allows. Breathing practices can be especially beneficial for children and adults with attention deficit hyperactivity. In our book, *Non-Drug Treatments for ADHD*, we describe breathing and other mind-body practices for ADHD.

How to Slow Down

Suppose you have really tried to do Coherent Breathing at five breaths per minute and even at six breaths per minute, but you just cannot slow your breath down. You feel too short of breath to go that slowly. Do not get discouraged. You simply need to slow your breathing down more gradually. Stephen Elliot's *Slow Down!* CD will help you to do this more comfortably. You may order the CD on his Web site, www.coherence.com, and as you listen to the CD you can follow the "Specific Instructions for Slowing Down" below.

The *Slow Down!* CD contains sixteen consecutive breathing rhythms, ranging from twenty breaths per minute to five breaths per minute. Each recording consists of a high note followed by a low note that repeats over and over again for the duration of the track. We suggest inhaling on the high note and exhaling on the low note. Toward the end of each note, you hear a chime. The chime signals that the note is about to end and that a change from inhalation to exhalation or from exhalation to inhalation is nearing.

Specific Instructions for Slowing Down

Step 1: Before you begin, sit comfortably for a moment. With a watch or clock, count the number of times you normally inhale or exhale per minute. Try not to change your current breathing pattern, just count the number of inhalations or exhalations. Record this number. We'll call it our "current breathing rate."

Step 2: Turn on the *Slow Down!* CD. Find the track that corresponds to your current breathing rate — for example, fifteen breaths per minute, and practice breathing at this rate for the duration of the track, about four minutes. This helps to develop a smooth, rhythmic breathing cycle at your current breathing rate.

Step 3: When that track ends, it will automatically step to the next track. When it does, begin inhaling and exhaling at this lower rate for the duration of this next track. Continue in this way for two or three tracks—for example, practicing at fifteen, fourteen, and thirteen breaths per minute.

Step 4: The next day, begin at your current breathing rate minus one, again practicing for two or three tracks — for example, fourteen, thirteen, and twelve breaths per minute. Continue in this way, with the ultimate goal of comfortably reaching five breaths per minute. Once you do, try to breathe at five breaths per minute all the time, circumstances permitting.

Here is an example of how to slow your breathing down if your current breathing rate is eighteen breaths per minute.

1. Day 1   Use tracks at eighteen, seventeen, and sixteen breaths per minute.
2. Day 2   Use tracks at seventeen, sixteen, and fifteen breaths per minute.
3. Day 3   Use tracks at sixteen, fifteen, and fourteen breaths per minute.

4. Day 4   Use tracks at fifteen, fourteen, and thirteen breaths per minute.

Continue to reduce the breath rate by one breath per minute each day until you are able to do five or six breaths per minute comfortably. If you are not able to get all the way down to five breaths per minute because of physical limitations, that is OK. For example, if your lowest possible breath rate is eight breaths per minute, you will still succeed in improving the balance of your stress-response system. Over time, with daily practice, you will probably become able to further reduce your breathing rate.

Body Scan Relaxation

Now that you are adept at Coherent Breathing, you're ready to move on to the body scan. At the completion of the breath practices, it is best not to immediately jump up and start dashing about doing things. In order to allow the practice to settle deeply into your system and to consolidate its beneficial effects, we advise ending with a brief relaxation period. You may choose to do any form of relaxation you like, such as meditation, visualization, or your own variation of the body scan. Some people find that this is an ideal time for deep prayer, because the mind is clear and the heart and spirit are especially open after the breathing practice. But first we would like to guide you through a basic body scan, using the *Healing Power of the Breath* CD. The instructions for doing a basic body scan are as follows.

Basic Body Scan

After ten minutes of Coherent Breathing, lie down and play track 8.

Closing your eyes and your mouth, breathe slowly and gently in the Coherent Breathing rhythm.

Continuing the Coherent Breathing and keeping your body still, direct your attention to the soles of your feet.

Let your attention linger on the soles of your feet for a few moments.

Direct your attention to the tops of your feet.

Let your attention linger on the tops of your feet for a few moments.

Direct your attention to your ankles.

Let your attention linger on your ankles.

Direct your attention to your knees.

Let your attention linger on your knees.

Direct your attention to your hips.

Let your attention linger on your hips.

Direct your attention to your belly.

Let your attention linger on your belly.

Direct your attention to your chest.

Let your attention linger on your chest.

Direct your attention to your hands.

Let your attention linger on your hands.

Direct your attention to the crooks of your arms, the inside of your elbow where it bends.

Let your attention linger on the crooks of your arms.

Direct your attention to your neck.

Let your attention linger on your neck.

Direct your attention to your face.

Let your attention linger on your face.

Direct your attention to your head.

Let your attention linger on your head.

Direct your attention to your whole body.

Let your attention linger on your whole body.

Now just relax and breathe naturally. Roll onto your right side and rest a few minutes.

Notice how you feel.

Body Scan with Pulse Awareness

Once you are able to do Coherent Breathing for fifteen minutes, you will be ready to do a body scan relaxation process and test the flexibility of your circulatory system. There are many kinds of body scans. In general, they involve focusing your attention on different parts of the body, usually starting with the feet and moving up to the head. This body scan is a little different in that it asks you to focus your attention on your pulse. For this you will want to be lying down comfortably. When you focus your attention on each location, stay with it there for at least ten seconds before moving to the next spot. If you have more time to practice, you can linger at each spot a bit longer, perhaps for thirty seconds. It is better not to distract your mind with counting the seconds. Focus your attention on the pulse. Take the time to read this section all the way through before beginning this practice.

Pulse Body Scan

Begin by turning on the Coherent Breathing track (track 2 on the CD), and then lie down.

Closing your eyes and your mouth, breathe slowly and gently in the Coherent Breathing rhythm for about fifteen minutes.

Continuing the Coherent Breathing and keeping your body still, direct your attention to the outside edge of your toes. Is it possible to feel your pulse there? Feel the pulse for at least ten seconds at each location.

Can you feel your pulse at your ankle?

Is it possible to feel your pulse behind your knee?

Can you feel your pulse where your legs join your body?

Is it possible to feel your pulse in your belly?

Can you feel your pulse in your chest?

Is it possible to feel your pulse in the tips and sides of your fingers?

Can you feel your pulse in the crook of your arm, the inside of your elbow where it bends?

Is it possible to feel your pulse in your neck, in your throat?

Can you feel your pulse in the lips?

Is it possible to feel your pulse at your temples, just beyond the tips of your eyebrows?

Now just relax and breathe naturally. Roll onto your right side and rest a few minutes. Notice how you feel.

How is it possible to feel the pulse in so many places where you never felt it before? You are able to feel the pulse because Coherent Breathing increases the elasticity of your blood vessels and the amplitude of the pulse wave. As the walls of the blood vessels become more flexible, they expand (balloon out) more with each pulse wave. So, as the blood flows through the arteries, instead of a little blip, it creates a palpable pulse. Now you are seeing for yourself one of the ways that Coherent Breathing increases the flexibility of your vascular system.

If you cannot feel your pulse in all these places, don't worry about it. With a little more practice, as you increase your heart rate variability, you will eventually be able to feel your pulse in many places. For now, just direct your attention to the different parts of your body, even if you cannot feel the pulse there. Just the act of directing the attention enhances the relaxing effect of the body scan.

As you continue to work on Coherent Breathing and doing the body scan in your day-to-day life, you will begin to feel recharged, rejuvenated, and more in harmony with your emotions. Essentially, you are taking the time to reconnect with your body in a gentler, more healing way. The breathing will seamlessly bring you back to the natural mental and emotional flexibility you had as a child, but with the direction and purpose you have as an adult. Over time, you may find that you feel calmer, more relaxed, and more aware of your body, your breath, and your mind.

2

Why Cats Purr

Resistance Breathing

> And only then did I understand
> It is Jeoffry—and every creature like him—
> Who can teach us how to praise—purring
> In their own language,
> Wreathing themselves in the living fire.
>
> —*Edward Hirsch, "Wild Gratitude"*

R esistance Breathing is any kind of breathing that creates resistance to the flow of air. Resistance can be created by pursing the lips, placing the tip of the tongue against the inside of the upper teeth, hissing through clenched teeth, tightening the throat muscles, partly closing the glottis, narrowing the space between the vocal cords, or using an external object such as breathing through a straw.

Why would we want to create airway resistance? For the same reason that cats purr. What happens when a cat purrs? The purring sound is created by the breath moving past a partial obstruction of the upper airway, creating a vibrational sound. This has several effects that stimulate the soothing part of the cat's nervous system. So the purring is not only a sound that expresses a state of relaxation, the purring is actually inducing the relaxation.

In the previous chapter we introduced you to the soothing, relaxing, restoring part of the nervous system, known to scientists as the parasympathetic nervous system. This counterbalances the activating, energy-burning part called the sympathetic nervous system. The activating part gets us ready to do things we need to do as well as to respond to threat or danger by releasing adrenaline, speeding up the heart, increasing the respiratory rate, raising the blood pressure, and redistributing blood flow to the muscles of the arms and legs. This get-ready-for-action system burns a lot of energy, releases free radicals (small particles that damage cells), and increases inflammatory processes. The soothing, recharging part, the parasympathetic system, slows down the heart, slows respiration, calms the mind, restores energy reserves, repairs cells, and reduces inflammation. We need both systems, but for a healthy mind and body, we need them to be in balance.

As you recall from chapter 1, Coherent Breathing refers to the respiratory rate of five breaths per minute. Resistance Breathing refers to various techniques used to create resistance to the flow of air and thereby enhance the effects of Coherent Breathing. Resistance Breathing slightly increases pressure in the lungs, which heightens stimulation of the parasympathetic system, the soothing, recharging part of the nervous system.[1] Also, when the respiratory muscles have to work harder against resistance, they become stronger over time. Taking slower and deeper breaths also opens more of the lungs' alveoli, the tiny air-filled sacs through which oxygen enters the blood and carbon dioxide is expelled. The results are healthier lungs and better oxygenation. This is especially important for people who are prone to respiratory infections, pneumonia, or who have had atelectasis (collapse of lung tissue).

Breath: Portal to the Mind-Body System

A major component of the stress-response system is the autonomic nervous system, which orchestrates the automatic, or involuntary, functions of the body, including the cardiovascular, respiratory, digestive, hormonal, glandular, and immune systems. An intricate communication network carries messages from the brain to the body in order to regulate these automatic functions, while messages from the body ascend to inform the brain of the moment-to-moment state of every part of the body. If there is anything amiss with our breathing, the brain needs to know quickly to take action immediately. For instance, if the airway is obstructed by a piece of food, the brain has only three or four minutes to respond and restore respiration for survival. So, respiratory messages have top priority when it comes to getting the brain's attention. Thus, feedback from the body has powerful effects on how the brain works, what we feel, what we think, how we interpret what is going on, our perceptions, the decisions we make, and how we respond emotionally and physically to everything we experience.[2]

Of all the automatic functions of the body, only one can be easily controlled voluntarily — breathing. By voluntarily changing the rate, depth, and pattern of breathing, we can change the messages being sent from the body's respiratory system to the brain.[3] In this way, breathing techniques provide a portal to the autonomic communication network through which we can, by changing our breathing patterns, send specific messages to the brain using the language of the body, a language the brain understands and to which it responds. Messages from the respiratory system have rapid, powerful effects on major brain centers involved in thought, emotion, and behavior.[4] For instance, if we feel anxious, just a few minutes of Coherent Breathing can calm our worried mind and foster more rational, rather than impulsive, decision-making.

Why do so many people enjoy singing and chanting? Of course, music can be beautiful, uplifting, and unifying. But singing and chanting are also forms of Resistance Breathing that stimulate the parasympathetic nervous system and thereby make us feel good. The musical sounds are created by contracting the vocal cords to create airway resistance as the breath passes through the larynx (voice box). Vocal music that requires the singer to prolong the notes on exhalation is a particularly effective breathing practice, as are vocalizations that induce internal vibrations. These techniques add to the stimulation of the soothing, recharging parts of the nervous system. They provide the optimal effect of feeling relaxed and at the same time energized.

Resistance Breathing

Simply breathing through the nose creates a little more resistance to airflow than breathing through the mouth. We are going to teach you two different kinds of breathing that further increase airway resistance and thereby induce more powerful effects: pursed lips and Ocean Breath. Pursing the lips is probably easier to learn, but it requires shifting from breathing in through the nose to breathing out through the lips with each breath. The second technique has many names, such as Ocean Breath, Victory Breath, Noisy Breath, and, in Sanskrit, *ujjayi* (meaning "victory over the mind through the breath"). But for our purposes we will call it Resistance Breathing (using capitals *R* and *B*). Most people can master Resistance Breathing with a little practice, and it lends itself more easily to more advanced practices.

You can begin Resistance Breathing as soon as you learn Coherent Breathing. Resistance Breathing will actually make it easier to control and slow the airflow to maintain the Coherent Breathing respiratory rate. However, we suggest that you begin using Resistance Breathing only for the first five minutes of your breath practices and then gradually, over the course of a week or two, increase the length of time until you are able to use it for the full twenty minutes. As in training any other muscle, it takes time to strengthen the throat muscles to maintain contraction over long periods of time without straining, tiring, or hoarseness.

Breathing with Pursed Lips

Bring the upper lip down toward the lower lip, leaving a small narrow opening. Breathe out slowly through the small space between your lips. As with other forms of resistance breathing, breathing with pursed lips will help stimulate the soothing part of your nervous system. In addition it will help slow the flow of air and make it easier for you to prolong your breath.

You may sit or lie down in a comfortable position. Close your eyes. When you breathe in, close your mouth, and breathe through your nose. When you breathe out, breathe through pursed lips. Practice slowly breathing in through your nose and out through pursed lips for five minutes or until you can do it easily and without thinking about it. Now it is time to combine pursed-lip breathing with Coherent Breathing.

Coherent Breathing with Pursed-Lip Breathing

- Closing your eyes, breathe in through your nose and out through pursed lips.
- Play the second track of the *Healing Power of the Breath* CD.
- Continue breathing slowly as you listen to the "Two Bells" chime.
- Breathe in through the nose on one tone.
- Breathe out through pursed lips on the next tone.
- Breathe slowly and gently with the Coherent Breathing rate.
- Remember to relax your face, neck, shoulders, and hands.
- If it is going smoothly and easily, continue for another ten minutes. When you are finished, just rest.
- Notice how your body feels. Notice the quality of your mind.

Resistance Breathing: Ocean Breath, or *Ujjayi*

We use the term *Resistance Breathing* to indicate Ocean Breath, or *ujjayi* ("victory over the mind through the breath"). This Resistance Breathing entails making a soft sound like the sound of the ocean heard inside a seashell by slightly tightening the muscles at the upper back of the throat. This is best learned from an instructor who can check and correct your technique. However, many people are able to learn just by listening to the sound. You will hear this ocean sound on track 3, Resistance Breathing, of the *Healing Power of the Breath* CD. Another way to learn to make the ocean sound is to begin with your mouth open. Breathing out, make the whispery sound *ahhhhh,* the sound that you make after quenching your thirst on a hot day. Repeat this *ahhhhhh* several times with your eyes closed while focusing your attention on the feelings in the muscles being tightened in the upper back part of your throat. Next, close your mouth and repeat the same sound, a sound like white noise.

Those who already have experience doing Resistance Breathing will be able to do it on both the in-breath and the out-breath. But if you have not done this type of breathing before, we recommend using it for the out-breath only. Most people have difficulty learning to do Resistance Breathing on the in-breath without a teacher listening to their efforts and coaching them into it. You will reap the benefits of Resistance Breathing even if you only do it during the exhale. If you want to also use it on the inhale, we suggest you take a live workshop rather than engender the stress and frustration of trying to do it on your own.

Resistance Breathing with Ocean (*Ujjayi*) Breath

- Listen to the Ocean Breath sound on the Resistance Breathing track.
- Close your eyes and your mouth. Try to make the same sound yourself, as you breathe out through your nose.

- Once you think you have it, try to maintain the sound from the very beginning to the very end of the out-breath. It should be a steady sound, like white noise.
- Now make the same sound but more softly and with less effort. It should be present throughout the out-breath but barely audible.
- With your eyes closed, breathe in and out through your nose, using Resistance Breathing on the out-breath.
- Play the second track of the *Healing Power of the Breath* CD.
- Continue breathing with the Coherent Breathing rate.
- Breathe slowly and gently with Resistance Breathing.
- Remember to relax your neck and shoulders.
- If it is going smoothly and easily, continue for another ten minutes. When you are finished, just rest.
- Notice how your body feels. Notice the quality of your mind.

Using the *Healing Power of the Breath* CD, practice Coherent Breathing with either pursed lips or Resistance Breathing (Ocean Breath) once or twice a day. During the next seven days increase your practice time to twenty minutes for at least one of the sessions each day. Within a week of daily practice, you will develop greater strength and control of the throat muscles, and Resistance Breathing will have become easy and almost automatic. If this breathing causes discomfort in your neck or throat, stop, rest, and begin again, breathing more gently. Resistance Breathing should be done without any straining. The sound can be quite soft. The more you do this practice, the more you will benefit.

When should you use Coherent Breathing and when should you use Resistance Breathing?

We suggest that at the beginning of your twenty-minute Coherent Breathing practice you use Resistance Breathing until your muscles tire, then let it go and just do Coherent Breathing. As you practice each day and your throat muscles become stronger, extend the length of time for Resistance Breathing until you can sustain it throughout the twenty-minute practice.

When you do Coherent Breathing at night you may get so relaxed and drowsy that you forget to continue Resistance Breathing. No problem. The goal is to become deeply relaxed, so just let go of the Resistance Breathing and let yourself float off to sleep.

Resistance Breathing in Survivors of Sexual Trauma

In general, breath practices can be extremely helpful for survivors of trauma (as we will discuss in chapter 4). However, some people who have been victims of sexual assault may feel uncomfortable learning Resistance Breathing. This may occur if the sound created during Resistance Breathing reminds the person of the heavy breathing of their abuser during the assault. If you are a survivor of sexual abuse, you may try to learn Resistance Breathing, but if it causes you to feel uncomfortable, just stop doing it. You will still be able to get great benefits from Coherent Breathing and the other practices. You may find that pursed-lip breathing is more comfortable for you. Later on, after you have been using the breath practices for a few months, you may have released enough of the trauma-related stress that you become able to undertake Resistance Breathing with less difficulty. Always notice how you are feeling and base your practice on what your system needs.

Obstacles to Resistance Breathing

Most people find it easiest to learn one thing at a time. We teach Coherent Breathing first, because until the muscles are trained, it can be tiring to do Resistance Breathing for twenty minutes, which means it can create stress — which is just what we don't want during the breathing. Furthermore, there are many situations in which breathing through the nose is easier and less conspicuous than breathing through pursed lips. For example, if you feel stressed at work, would you rather keep pursing your lips or breathe inconspicuously through your nose? Once you become proficient in Ocean Breathing, you will be able to do it in any situation without anyone noticing.

When Resistance Breathing Hurts the Throat

If you are only doing Resistance Breathing for five minutes as a beginner and if your throat is hurting, then you are probably straining yourself by doing it too loudly or too forcefully. Remember, the sound does not have to be loud. It can be barely audible, and the breathing should be slow, gentle, and even. People make different sounds when first learning to do Resistance Breathing. We have heard everything: snoring, grunting, wheezing, gagging, and unrecognizable gravelly sounds. But in fact, what you are trying to achieve is just a soft, even sound, like ocean waves gently breaking on the shore.

Trying Too Hard

Pamela is a good example of what can happen when a person tries too hard. No matter where she went, what she did, or who she talked to, Pamela reacted to every situation with such severe anxiety and body tension that she became exhausted. She refused to take medication, because she believed that would make her symptoms worse. Pamela's therapist referred her to us, suggesting that she learn breath practices to reduce her incessant worrying. We taught her Coherent Breathing and Resistance Breathing, and gave her instructions to practice every day and return in two weeks. Upon returning, Pamela complained that the breathing was of no help at all, a waste of time, though she had done it every single day. We asked her to show us how she was doing the breathwork. Pamela sat on the edge of the chair, scrunched up her face, and clenched her hands. As she inhaled she pulled her shoulders up to her ears, and as she exhaled she slammed her shoulders back down, her breath forced out in short, choppy grunts. No wonder it wasn't working. Apparently, Pamela infused everything she did with this kind of tension.

For instance, when she was supposed to take a leisurely walk through her charming gardens, it became a forced march. Pamela needed to first work on why she was driving herself like a drill sergeant. She needed to learn to let herself relax enough to benefit from the breath practices.

Get Closer with Resistance Breathing

Just for fun, try synchronizing Resistance Breathing with your cat's purring—you will have one more way to communicate with your pet. You can also use Coherent Breathing and Resistance Breathing with your partner. Couples who breathe together find it enhances feelings of closeness. It's also nice to be able to fall asleep around the same time. Remember, the couple that breathes together makes Zs together.

As with purring, singing your favorite songs, and chanting, Resistance Breathing has a place in your daily life. It can become a part of your most cherished activities simply because it helps you to relax, to be fully present and aware, and to enhance your sense of peace, joy, and connection to yourself and to others.

3

A Balancing Act

Breath Moving, the Total Breath, the Complete Practice

> Moving the breath relaxes and refreshes, like an internal massage
> and shower.
>
> —*Dr. Richard P. Brown*

In Breath Moving we use our imagination to move our breath and
awareness to different parts of the body. This method improves the circulation of energy through the nervous system and improves blood flow.
Many mind-body traditions use a variety of practices to increase energy
flow. Some Eastern traditions consider blocks to the flow of energy to be
the root cause of illness. They view mind-body practices as a way to open
chakras (energy centers) and dissolve blockages in the body's channels so
that energy and vital substances can circulate more freely. Western science
has just begun to study many of these techniques, and therefore we have
much to learn about how they exert their effects. Nevertheless, you will
notice definite changes in your mind and body as you practice moving
your breath.

If you have asthma, you may experience some difficulty breathing
when you try to do Coherent Breathing alone. If this occurs, start your

practice with Breath Moving to open the airways. Once the airways are open, slow your breath rate gradually until you are able to follow the pacing tones on the *Healing Power of the Breath* CD that accompanies this book. Always begin your practice with Breath Moving and continue Breath Moving throughout. Also, it may be easier for you to start with track 10 at six breaths per minute on the CD rather than track 2 or 8 at five breaths per minute.

You may have found that when you do Coherent Breathing and Resistance Breathing your mind tends to wander. Breath Moving will help to keep your mind focused on the breath practices. It thereby increases concentration while at the same time maintaining a more open, rather than rigidly narrowed, focus. In this way, your attention has an inner focus while remaining open and receptive. This expands your awareness.

The ancient roots of Breath Moving are in China. Forms of it are also evident in Hawaiian mind-body practices and in qigong. Ancient Hawaiian Huna healing uses *piko-piko* breathing to move energy between the naval and the crown of the head. The technique of moving the breath was developed to a high degree by Russian Christian Orthodox Hesychast monks around the eleventh century. The monks used the practice in preparation for the Jesus Prayer to attain deep states of prayer and meditation. Because the practices were secret, they were never written down. At that time, the holy Russian warriors were defending their realm against invaders. The monks taught their breath techniques to the holy warriors to make them more resilient, so that they would sustain less damage when attacked in battle. In addition, the techniques heightened their awareness, a vital capacity in combat. They also believed that these practices increased awareness of the spiritual aspects of everyday existence. Traces of these practices have remained as part of the training for elite Russian Special Forces soldiers. A veteran of this Russian military training, Vladimir Vasiliev, moved to Canada and in 1993 founded a martial arts school of Systema that has developed an international following. Traditionally taught as a mind-body-soul method of health and conditioning, Systema employs intense breathing methods as the foundation of its combat training.[1]

Breath Moving: Beginning Practice

The Breath Moving methods in this book are derived from the study and practice of Japanese and Chinese martial arts, Hesychast monks, Russian fitness training, qigong, and written descriptions of Systema training. The breath can be moved in myriad circuits and directions. Here you will learn the first two basic circuits. The more advanced circuits are taught in our Breath~Body~Mind workshops.

Breath Moving: The First Two Circuits

You may sit or lie down in a comfortable position.
- Close your eyes and your mouth.
- Breathe in and out through your nose.
- Play track 4 of the *Healing Power of the Breath* CD.
- Breathe in through the nose on one tone.
- Breathe out through the nose on the next tone.
- Repeat breathing in on one tone and out on the following tone.
- Breathe slowly and gently with the Coherent Breathing rate.
- Remember to relax your face, neck, shoulders, and hands.

Basic Breath Moving, Circuit 1

- On the next tone, as you breathe in, imagine you are moving your breath to the top of your head.
- As you breathe out, imagine you are moving your breath to the base of your spine, your perineum, your sit bones.
- Each time you breathe in, move the breath to the top of the head.
- Each time you breathe out, move the breath to the base of the spine.
- Breathe in this circuit for ten cycles.

Basic Breath Moving, Circuit 2

- On the next tone, as you breathe in, imagine you are moving your breath to the top of your head.
- As you breathe out, imagine you are moving your breath down through your body and out through the soles of your feet, like a bubbling stream.
- Each time you breathe in, imagine the breath coming in through the soles of your feet and moving up your legs and body to the top of your head.
- Each time you breathe out, move the breath down and out through the soles of the feet.
- Breathe in this circuit for ten cycles.

Basic Breath Moving, Repeat Circuit 1

- On the next tone, as you breathe in, imagine you are moving your breath to the top of your head.
- As you breathe out, imagine you are moving your breath to the base of your spine.
- Each time you breathe in, move the breath to the top of the head.
- Each time you breathe out, move the breath to the base of the spine.
- Breathe in this circuit for ten cycles.

Rest the Breath

- Let your breath rest as you continue to breathe in the Coherent Breathing rate.
- Notice how your body feels. Notice the quality of your mind.

We recommend that you practice basic Breath Moving every day for five to ten minutes while doing your Coherent Breath practice. When you can do it smoothly and easily, you will be ready for the Total Practice.

Always begin and end with circuit 1, from the top of the head to the base of the spine. You can vary the number of times you do each circuit before switching to the other. For example: circuit 1 ten times, circuit 2 ten times, circuit 1 ten times, circuit 2 ten times, and so on.

Obstacles to the Practice of Breath Moving

Most people find it easy to learn Breath Moving. However, here are two obstacles you might encounter and ways to resolve them.

Difficulty Visualizing the Breath Moving

Some people find it difficult to imagine or visualize the breath moving inside their body. Visualization is helpful but not essential. First try different ways of visualizing the breath as an energy flow or as a stream of water or feel it as a breeze moving through you. If you have difficulty visualizing, just focus your attention completely on the place where you want the breath to go. Become intensely aware of that place. For example, to move the energy to the top of your head, focus on feeling either the top of your head, your scalp, or the hair at the top of your head. Then focus your attention on the base of your spine, the feeling where it meets the floor or the chair. Continue moving your attention to the focal points of each circuit. This will work even without actual visualization. With practice it becomes easier.

Feeling Activated Instead of Calm

While most people derive calm feelings from Breath Moving, for some it is more activating and energizing. If you respond to Breath Moving by feeling activated, then use this technique in the morning and during the day to refresh and energize yourself. For you, it would be better not to use it at night. Instead, at night use only Coherent Breathing and Resistance Breathing to prepare for sleep.

Total Breath = Coherent Breathing + Resistance + Breath Moving

Once you have mastered Breath Moving at the Coherent Breathing rate and you are able to perform it smoothly and without strain, you will be ready to learn the Total Breath. Each form of breathing we add to your practice increases the stimulation of the soothing, recharging, healing part of your nervous system. While these breath practices have traditionally been used separately, we combine them into one Total Breath practice in order to intensely activate the parasympathetic system and create the most powerful effects on the stress-response system in the shortest possible time. The Total Breath practice starts with Coherent Breathing, then adds Breath Moving, and then Resistance Breathing, combining these into one transformative practice. Instead of taking an hour to do three breath practices, you will be able to do all three together in about twenty minutes, as described in the instructions that follow.

The Total Breath

You may sit or lie down in a comfortable position.
- Close your eyes and your mouth.
- Breathe in and out through your nose.
- Play the second track of the *Healing Power of the Breath* CD.
- Breathe in through the nose on one tone.
- Breathe out through the nose on the other tone.
- Breathe slowly and gently with the Coherent Breathing rate.
- Remember to relax your neck and shoulders.

Basic Breath Moving, Circuit 1

- On the next tone, as you breathe in, imagine you are moving your breath up to the top of your head.

- As you breathe out, imagine you are moving your breath down to the base of your spine.
- Each time you breathe in, move the breath to the top of the head.
- Each time you breathe out, move the breath to the base of the spine.
- Breathe with this circuit for five cycles.

Total Breath

- As you do the Breath Moving circuit, begin to use Resistance Breathing.
- When you feel comfortable using Total Breath in circuit 1, begin using it in circuit 2.
- Alternate about ten rounds of Total Breath in circuit I with ten rounds in circuit 2.
- If you begin to tire from the Resistance Breathing, let it go and just use Breath Moving with Coherent Breathing. You can do the Resistance Breathing for short periods of time until you develop the stamina to use it throughout the practice. It is most important to do the breathwork in a way that is relaxed, comfortable, and without any strain.

The Complete Practice: Movement, Breathing, and Meditation

Most traditional mind-body practices have multiple components. For example, classical yoga has what are called the Eight Limbs for complete mental, physical, and spiritual development. These include movement, breathing, meditation, and the practice of character virtues such as honesty, nonharming, and right living. Just as we need variety in our diets, we also need variety in our mind-body practices. The more we find ways to release tension, balance our nervous systems, and harmonize our personal lives, the more likely we are to achieve healthy changes. If you were to choose just one type of practice, you could choose the breathing you have learned so far, and just doing that every day would bring about positive emotional and physical changes over time. If you have the time to do a little more, however, we would suggest that you begin your practice with five to ten minutes of physical movement and end your practice with five minutes of relaxation or meditation. If you already have a meditation practice, you will find that by doing the Total Breath first, you will be able to quiet your mind and enter more smoothly and deeply into your meditation. The ideal sequence would be movement, breathing, and relaxation or meditation.

In chapter 1 you learned the body scan, a basic relaxation practice to follow Coherent Breathing. For the movement segment of your practice you can use any kind of slow movements, such as yoga, qigong, tai chi, or a basic set of warm-up muscle and tendon stretches. The warm-up could include head rolls, shoulder rolls, stretching the calves, heels, and thighs, spinal stretches, extending the arms upward and to the sides, and so forth. If you combine slow Resistance Breathing with these movements it will enhance the stretching and increase the benefits in the same amount of time. Chapter 5 will introduce you to additional techniques, each with their own benefits. The general rule is to inhale with rising movements and to exhale with descending movements. Here are two examples of how to combine Resistance Breathing with movement.

Resistance Breathing with Head Rolls

- Stand with your feet shoulder-width apart. Straighten your head, keeping your chin level, and relax your knees. Imagine your head being pulled by a string up toward the sky. Imagine your feet planted solidly on the ground, growing deep roots into the earth.
- Allow your head to tilt forward until your chin rests on your chest. Slowly rotate your head in a circle to the right as you slowly inhale.

- When you are halfway around and your head is tilted to the back, begin to exhale slowly with Resistance Breathing as you continue to rotate your head around to the left and bring it back to the center of your chest.
- Repeat this rotation to the right five times and then rotate to the left five times.
- As you rotate your head, if you notice pain and stiffness in a particular position, pause and take several slow breaths while you imagine the breath moving through the painful point.
- Notice the change in how your neck feels.

Resistance Breathing with Shoulder Rolls

- Stand with your feet shoulder-width apart. Straighten your head, keeping your chin level, and relax your knees. Imagine your head being pulled on a string up toward the sky. Imagine your feet planted solidly on the ground, growing roots deep into the earth.
- Slowly rotate your shoulders in a circle by bringing them forward and up as you slowly inhale.
- When your shoulders get to the top of the circle halfway around, exhale slowly with Resistance Breathing as you continue to rotate your shoulders around to the back.
- Repeat this rotation from forward to back five times, or more if you wish.
- Slowly rotate your shoulders in a circle by pushing them toward your back and then bringing them upward as you slowly inhale.
- When your shoulders get to the top of the circle halfway around, exhale slowly with Resistance Breathing as you continue to rotate your shoulders forward and down.
- Repeat this rotation from back to front back five times, or more if you like.
- Relax and notice how your shoulders feel.

Arm Raising to Stretch the Spine

- Stand with your feet shoulder-width apart. Straighten your head, keeping your chin level, and relax your knees. Imagine your head being pulled on a string up toward the sky. Imagine your feet planted solidly on the ground, growing deep roots into the earth.
- Raise your right arm slowly, palm facing inward, with your fingers pointed toward the sky. Your left arm should hang at your side with your fingers pointing toward the earth. Keeping your spine straight, inhale slowly as you reach your right arm higher toward the sky while you stretch your left arm down toward the earth. Exhale slowly with Resistance Breathing each time you release the stretch. Repeat this five times. Lower your right arm.
- Relax and become aware of the difference in how your right side feels in comparison with your left side.
- Raise your left arm slowly, palm facing inward with your fingers pointed toward the sky. Your right arm should hang at your side with your fingers pointing toward the earth. Keeping your spine straight, inhale slowly as you reach your left arm higher toward the sky while you stretch your right arm down toward the earth. Exhale slowly with Resistance Breathing each time you release the stretch. Repeat this five times. Lower your left arm.
- Relax and notice the change in how your body feels.

Additional Movements

If you have time to do more body stretches, just continue to use the breathing and pause after completing each movement to notice changes in how your body feels. This helps to teach your brain to listen to your body and improves your awareness of subtle changes. Use slow breathing with or without Resistance Breathing to enhance stretches for your neck, back, trunk, arms, and legs, as well as for joint rotations. While doing joint rotations imagine your breath moving into and through the joint. This will help improve your range of motion and reduce any joint pains you may be having. If you want to learn more stretches or yoga postures, you could participate in a class or follow a DVD program. For people who have never done yoga, it would be better to take some classes with a certified yoga teacher who could help assure that the movements are done correctly and without strain. In the resources section at the end of the book, you will find some suggestions for good programs.

Occupational Hazards

Every job has its pluses and minuses. Many jobs probably require the repeated use of certain sets of muscles or some degree of stress on your joints. This can lead to problems such as chronic pain, wearing down of joints, headaches, back and neck problems, or the dreaded carpal tunnel syndrome. Whether from computer work, physical labor, or athletic activities, it is likely that at some time you will experience musculoskeletal problems, inflamed tendons, muscle spasms, or aches and pains. Below we look at examples of situations in which slow Resistance Breathing with muscle stretching and joint rotations can help to prevent muscle and joint problems from developing or help to relieve ailments that have already occurred.

Computer Blues

Even if your job does not require much keyboarding, if you are like most people you probably spend a good deal of time on your home computer. Once you become absorbed in whatever has captured your attention, you lose track of time. Only when your neck starts to hurt or you feel that twinge in your lower back do you realize how long you have been sitting without moving. Cyberspace has mesmerized your mind to such an extent that your brain has stopped listening to your body—until your body shouts out with a pang strong enough to break the trance. The body posture of people who spend the greatest number of hours every day sitting at a computer may even gel into a state of contraction in which the head extends forward, the shoulders and back are hunched, the elbows stay partially bent, and the movements become stiff. Stress from work or academic pressures also contributes to the build-up of muscle tension.

Whenever you sit at a desk or computer, it is best to take short breaks at least once an hour to do head and shoulder rotations. Head rolls and shoulder rotations are an excellent way to relieve tension in the neck, shoulders, and back. You can use Resistance Breathing while slowly rotating your neck and then your shoulders five times each way as you learned above. If there is residual tension, you can repeat the same sequence and do it more frequently. This will help prevent muscle tension from building up in the neck and upper back. If you become so absorbed that you forget to take breaks, use a small timer set for one hour to remind you to stop, stretch, and listen to your body.

Carpal Tunnel Syndrome

While carpal tunnel syndrome used to be a problem that mostly occurred in people whose jobs involved extreme overuse of their hands, such as dentists and musicians, in the computer era it has become a much more common condition. Overuse of the hands in keyboarding can lead to inflammation of tendons in the lower arm and wrist. The inflamed tendons enlarge, compressing the carpal tunnel, a passageway containing nerve fibers. The result is pain that may require wearing a hand and wrist support or possibly surgery to reopen the tunnel. Overuse causes tendons to tighten and contract. Tendons need to be repeatedly stretched to keep them healthy and flexible. One method to keep wrist joints and tendons flexible is the use of wrist rotations combined with slow Resistance Breathing and Breath Moving.

Wrist Rotations

- Stand with your feet shoulder-width apart. Straighten your head, keeping your chin level and relaxing your knees. Imagine your head being pulled on a string up toward the sky. Imagine your feet planted solidly on the ground, growing deep roots into the earth.
- Raise both arms, holding them straight out in front of you. Curve your fingers toward your palms to form cup shapes and maintain the cups throughout the movements.
- Rotate both wrists and hands slowly in circles turning outward so that the right hand is rotating toward the right and the left hand is rotating toward the left. As you rotate, do slow Resistance Breathing and focus your attention and your breath inside your wrists. Repeat ten times.
- Rotate both hands and wrists slowly toward the inside so that the right hand is rotating toward the left and the left hand is rotating toward the right.
- Shake both hands for a few seconds. Relax and notice the change in how your hands feel.

First Responders

Responding to emergencies is extremely demanding both physically and psychologically. In addition to everyday emergencies such as accidents, first responders are also called upon to deal with natural disasters such as floods, wildfires, and earthquakes as well as man-made disasters such as terrorist attacks, oil spills, and nuclear accidents. After years of doing such grueling work, first responders develop the same types of joint and muscle injuries that occur in military personnel. And like combat soldiers, their bodies absorb and hold the stress of witnessing victims being injured or killed.

Through our involvement with a nonprofit organization called Serving Those Who Serve, we have had the privilege of working with first responders and Ground Zero workers who have not fully recovered from the intense work, stress, and toxic exposures following the September 11, 2001, terrorist attacks on the World Trade Center in New York City. We have been struck by the discipline and the stoicism of these individuals. They have not complained about their injuries but we have heard their groans and their sighs of relief as they learned to rotate and breathe through their painful joints. Over time, with regular practice, old injuries have begun to heal. We have seen similar responses in our work with military personnel, both those on active duty and veterans.

Sports Injuries

Whatever sport you play, you have probably developed a strain, a pain, or a crick somewhere in your body. Wherever you notice an injury developing, you can use the same method of rotating and flexing with Resistance Breathing, Breath Moving through the injury, and focused attention. These exercises help to lubricate the joints, preventing wear and tear; they stretch the tendons, improve circulation, reduce inflammation, and help to maintain flexibility. If you love sports, you will love the results.

Moving Forward

Let's briefly review what you have learned about the core breathing practices, the Total Breath, and the Complete Practice. The core breathing practices are Coherent Breathing, Resistance Breathing, and Breath Moving. Coherent Breathing uses the *Healing Power of the Breath* CD track to maintain a rate of five to six breaths per minute. Resistance Breathing creates a soft ocean sound by partial obstruction of the flow of air. During Breath Moving, attention is focused on moving the breath through body areas that need healing or on creating circuits that move the breath imaginatively between two places in the body—for example, between the top of the head and the base of the spine. The Total Breath is achieved by combining all three breath forms — Coherent Breathing, Resistance Breathing, and Breath Moving — to produce the Total Breath. Three breath forms are combined into one not only to save time but also to boost the therapeutic effects on stress resilience and the body's regulatory systems.

Complete Practice includes a sequence of movement, breathing, and meditation. In the next chapter, we will focus on breath practices for stress, job burnout, anxiety, phobias, depression, trauma, and mass disasters. In the subsequent chapters you will discover additional breathing techniques that produce different effects, and you will also learn how to use these practices to deal with many different conditions, circumstances, and relationships. The healing power of the breath will help you overcome negative emotions, freeing you to be more creative, more connected, and more loving. If, after reading through this book, you still have unanswered questions, you are welcome to contact us at www.haveahealthymind.com and we will do our best to respond.

4

The Winds of Change

Breath Practices for Stress, Insomnia, Anxiety, Phobias,
Burnout, Depression, Trauma, and Mass Disasters

When the mind is agitated, change the pattern of the breath.

—*Patanjali*, Yoga Sutras

Now that you have learned the core breathing practices, they are yours forever. No one can take them from you. They will never run out, run down, or expire. They belong to you. So, what will you do with them? When you are at home, in school, at work, or at play, there are infinite ways to use the breath to enrich every moment of your life. Breathing can alleviate negative feelings, such as fear, anxiety, frustration, anger, depression, self-blame, confusion, restlessness, and physical discomforts. With regular practice over time breathwork can bring improvements in physical health, endurance, and resilience. But breathing is not just a treatment for life's ills; it can also enhance pleasurable and creative activities such as musical performance, writing, team sports, or just being with nature. Breath practices nurture positive emotions, loving feelings, compassion, our sense of connection with what is meaningful in life, and our sense of bonding with others.

In this chapter we will look at how breath practices can help deal with common stress-related problems. We will also explore the role of breathing in the prevention of and recovery from serious illness, trauma, and mass disasters. Scientific studies and individual stories will be included.

Stress and Negative Emotions

Stress occurs whenever we have to adapt to change. Small amounts of stress are good for us: through adapting successfully to stressful situations, we become stronger and more competent. However, excess stress, stress that is beyond our ability to master, can lead us into a cycle of negative emotions such as worry, fear, and anxiety. When this continues without relief, it can become a whirlwind of frustration, anger, exhaustion, self-loathing, and depression.

How often do we have to adapt to change? Pretty much every day. Every day something changes in our personal life, in our family, in our body, in our portfolio, in our community, in our world. So, every day, we have to digest a certain amount of stress. This is why we recommend doing the Total Breath for at least twenty minutes every morning—to start the day with a balanced, resilient stress-response system. In this way, whatever problems come your way, you will respond with the calmness and clarity you need to make good decisions and finish the day feeling positively about what you have accomplished.

Mary-Anne, an education consultant for a large inner-city school, discovered these benefits shortly after learning the breath practices in one of our workshops. She wrote to let us know what had happened in her life in the weeks after the workshop. She said that she felt amazingly rested and refreshed after the workshop and that she wanted to use the breath in working with clients. The next day there had been a crisis at the school and an ambulance had to be called to take a student away. The classroom teacher was reeling from the shock of what she'd experienced with a deeply disturbed second grader. Mary-Anne met her in the corridor, and, seeing her anguish, took her aside for a few minutes to breathe using the five-breaths-per-minute Coherent Breathing technique she had learned at the workshop. Soon the teacher gave in to the relief of tears and then began talking about how she was feeling. She had been headed straight back to her classroom to stoically face the class and the rest of her day without time to cope with her own pain and the impact of her experience. Her whole body responded quickly to the breathing, enabling her to release some of the shock and tension. Afterward, she felt calmer and ready to handle her class.

Mary-Anne said she continued to practice the breathing, achieving states of deep relaxation. The following week, two of her school principals were in a panic about impending state visits, and she had to work long into the night to assist with restructuring plans and compliance documents in preparation. Coherent Breathing helped her stay focused and calm during that week of sleep deprivation. She felt that the periods of deep breathing helped her face the atmosphere of panic and fear (about possible school closure or dismissal), resist being overwhelmed by the fear, and steadily get the job done. She found herself using Coherent Breathing on the subway train, in the office and at home. Mary-Anne was able to use the breath practices immediately to help herself, her coworkers, her principals, and her schools. You can imagine the ripple effects—like a pebble tossed into a pond—as she spread her calmness to the teacher who carried it to the students in her classroom. She also helped relieve some of the stress affecting the principals and other members of the staff throughout those stress-filled offices.

You, too, will find that once you have learned Coherent Breathing you will immediately be able to use it to deal with a range of stressful situations, whether you are at home, at work, in the dentist's chair, or traveling. Moreover, you can share the benefits by teaching those around you a simple way to deal with the stressors in their lives. Once you establish an inner calm, you will transmit it naturally to others.

Breathing for Sleep Time

Steve could not get to sleep at night. As soon as his head hit the pillow, a switch went on in his brain. Instead of sleeping, he would lie there thinking, thinking, thinking. The more he tried to shut down his thoughts, the more they kept going . . . thoughts about mistakes of the past . . . thoughts about tomorrow's tasks . . . thoughts about not being able to stop his thoughts . . . fears of being unable to sleep . . . worries about being tired in the morning . . . frustration . . . anger . . . and so on for hours. He began to dread bedtime. Steve's doctor had offered him sleep medication, but he was afraid of becoming dependent on pills for sleep. His doctor advised him to consult a psychiatrist.

When Steve first came to Dr. Gerbarg's office he appeared tired and depressed. However, when she explained that he could learn to use breathing practices instead of taking medication, he perked up and agreed to try. Being highly motivated, Steve paid close attention and followed instructions well. Within a few minutes, he was well into the Coherent Breathing rhythm. His belly rose and fell naturally as he allowed himself to relax. He appeared to be on the edge of sleep, but he was aware enough to keep pace with the bell tones. Dr. Gerbarg did not want to disturb him, but the session was nearly over. She gently suggested that he return to normal breathing and open his eyes, but he didn't want to. Steve longed to hold on to the precious feeling of deep relaxation. She told him that now that he knew how to do Coherent Breathing, he would be able to give himself deep relaxation whenever he wanted. Finally he opened his eyes and said, "I can do that." When Steve returned for a follow-up visit, he looked well-rested. Using the *Respire-1* CD to pace his breathing enabled him to drift off to sleep at night. On his own, he had started using Coherent Breathing on and off during the day to stay relaxed during stressful situations. Steve learned Resistance Breathing and went on to take a Breath~Body~Mind workshop to go even deeper into breathwork.

Insomnia: Thinking Instead of Sleeping

Stress, anxiety, and thinking too much can all interfere with sleep. In addition to its calming effect, coherent breathing also turns off the worry centers of the brain.

Anxiety: I'm Worried Now, but I Won't Be Worried Long

Have you ever noticed that people who think a lot tend to worry a lot? The overactive mind can be a blessing or a curse. It is wonderful to be able to think through a problem, to handle details, to come up with answers. But when we get caught in excessive worry, the mind becomes a hamster running and running on a wheel that goes nowhere. Sometimes anxiety or insecurity can start the worry circuit, as though we believe that by worrying we can prevent a calamity. Once it gets going, it can be very difficult to stop, as was the case with a patient named Janice.

Janice was a very successful lawyer, but she had a tendency to worry about her son. Whenever she was aware that he was having a problem, her mind would jump onto the worry wheel. Whenever the phone rang, she would feel a pang of anxiety. She came to Dr. Gerbarg for help because the worry was causing anxiety and tension resulting in difficulty sleeping, daytime fatigue, and painful tension in her neck and shoulders. She explained her problem, "I know my worries are irrational, but I can't stop them. Telling myself not to worry doesn't stop it. Other people tell me not to worry. That doesn't help, either." Janice did not want to become dependent on antianxiety medications, which had caused problems for her in the past. Antidepressants made her feel jittery and disinterested in sex. She had been in counseling once a week for two years. Although she found it helpful to talk with her counselor, so far the sessions had not stopped her from worrying. She was looking for another approach.

Janice learned the Total Breath in one therapy session. Eager for results, she practiced twenty minutes faithfully every day for two weeks. At her next session, she came into the office smiling and looking far more relaxed than she had before. Janice described what had happened. "I did the breathing twice a day exactly as you told me and that helped me feel more relaxed," she reported. "I stopped tensing up whenever the phone rang. When I noticed myself starting to worry, I immediately started to do the Resistance Breathing, slowly, around the Coherent Breathing rate. The breathing stopped the worrying thoughts. Now I can get to sleep every night just by listening to the *Healing Power of the Breath* CD and breathing with the chimes. I don't get to the end because I fall asleep within the first ten minutes."

One of the ways that Coherent Breathing and Resistance Breathing work is by turning off the "worry centers" of the brain. These forms of breathing stimulate the vagus nerves, the main pathways of the parasympathetic nervous system. These pathways ascend to relay stations in the brainstem and extend via the thalamus to the cerebral cortex, where they quiet the excess thinking activity. At the same time, other branches of the pathway enter the centers of emotion regulation in the prefrontal cortex and in the limbic system, including the amygdala and hippocampus, where they help reduce anxiety and emotional overreactivity.[1] The tendency to calm both the intellect and the emotions may account for the rapid effects of these breath practices in reducing negative thoughts and emotions, such as excessive worry and anxiety.

Specific Phobias

Phobias are specific fears that are so intense they can significantly impair a person's ability to function in daily life. For example, people with claustrophobia may become anxious or have panic attacks in enclosed spaces such as elevators, stairwells, rooms, stores, or buildings. Fear of flying is another common phobia. But the most widespread phobia of all is fear of public speaking. Human beings are afraid of appearing foolish in front of a crowd, afraid of public humiliation. This can be especially problematic for teachers who must speak before a classroom every day or for people who must make presentations in the course of their work. Fear of public speaking can affect career choices.

Dr. Gerbarg's Fear of Public Speaking

I was one of those people who feared public speaking. Talking in front of a class was nerve-racking, because the anxiety made it hard to collect my thoughts to remember what I was going to say, and it made my knees weak. It isn't easy to do a good presentation when you feel spaced-out from anxiety. Then there was the fear that someone in the audience might ask a question that I could not answer. I didn't want to look like an idiot in front of everyone. One time the anxiety was so intense that my jaw locked, and I had to complete a presentation through clenched teeth. That was the end of my public speaking for the next fifteen years. The fear of having to deliver lectures was one of the factors that led me to relinquish a promising academic career and plunge right into pure clinical work.

Every year for over ten years, my husband, Dr. Richard Brown, and I have taught full-day courses on complementary and integrative medicine at the annual meetings of the American Psychiatric Association. Because we work closely on all research and writing projects, he wanted me to present some of the lectures. Each year when it came time for me to speak, the anxiety would well up. I'd shake my head no and let him deliver all of our lectures.

After I began doing daily breathing practices, my husband coached me on lecturing, but that year when the time came, I still avoided it. I started the breathing practices primarily to improve my physical endurance, with no expectation that they would affect my speaking phobia. So it was quite a surprise to us both the following year when it was my turn to lecture. He looked at me quizzically to see if I was ready to speak, and, instead of saying no, without thinking, I stepped up to the microphone and addressed the audience. I actually had fun lecturing. It had taken almost two years of breathwork to overcome that phobia. Now I look forward to giving lectures, and I especially enjoy answering people's questions.

The effects of anxiety and worry on performance can be devastating in the workplace, on the playing field, in the theater or concert hall, in any public performance setting, and in the privacy of the bedroom. Everyone has had some kind of anxiety. When it isn't paralyzing, anxiety can actually enhance performance by increasing energy and heightening awareness. However, when anxiety interferes with clear thinking, causes us to tense up, disturbs the fluidity of our movements, or changes our experience from pleasure to torment, then it undermines our best efforts. In chapter 7 we will explore in depth the use of breath practices to overcome performance anxiety and blocks to achievement. Even for people who have little or no anxiety, breath practices can be used to enhance physical, mental, and social performance.

Generalized Anxiety Disorder

People with generalized anxiety disorder (GAD) suffer from excessive anxiety and worry more days than not.[2] They may also experience restlessness, fatigue, irritability, difficulty concentrating, muscle tension, or sleep problems. A disorder that lasts for six months or more, GAD causes significant distress or impairs how the person functions in social situations, at school, or at work. In many cases medication and years of therapy bring only partial relief.

The S.T.A.R.T. Clinic for Mood and Anxiety Disorders, associated with the University of Toronto, is a tertiary care center, meaning that it specializes in treating more severe GAD patients who have not responded to multiple attempts by other care providers. In addition to serious GAD, most of their patients have coexisting diagnoses such as panic disorder, social phobia, obsessive compulsive disorder, PTSD, or depression. Monica Vermani, PhD, is a clinical psychologist and is certified to teach yoga, cognitive behavior therapy, and mindfulness-based cognitive behavior therapy (MBCBT). She knew about our work and introduced us to the S.T.A.R.T. Clinic director, Dr. Martin Katzman. Always looking for innovative ways to help his patients, Dr. Katzman offered to do scientific studies of breathing techniques as an adjunct to standard treatment.

The first open study used Sudarshan Kriya Yoga (SKY), a six-day program of yoga, breath practices, and meditation developed by Sri Sri Ravi Shankar, cofounder of the International Association for Human Values, a large NGO affiliated with the United Nations. The thirty-one patients who completed this study had already been treated with CBT, MBCT, and numerous medications, but were still symptomatic. Participants in the SKY workshop experienced significant improvements on tests of anxiety, including the Hamilton Anxiety Scale (HAM-A), within six weeks and the improvements persisted when they were retested six months later. Based on HAM-A scores, the response was 73 percent and the remission rate was 41 percent.[3]

After the first study, we developed a two-day program, the Breath~Body~Mind workshop, in order to reduce the training time and make the practices safer and more adaptable to different clinical populations. The second open study with Dr. Katzman and Dr. Vermani used Breath~Body~Mind to treat a similar group of twenty-seven GAD patients. Again, the response was robust, showing significant improvements in measures of anxiety and depression at the six-week testing, including the Beck Anxiety Inventory, the Beck Depression Inventory II, the anxiety sensitivity index, the Pittsburgh Sleep Quality Index, the Sheehan Disability Scale, and the Penn State Worry Questionnaire.[4]

Mass Disasters

Most mass disasters are beyond our comprehension. It may be the enormity of the devastation, the unfathomable human suffering, the sheer unfairness, or the fact that they are often unexpected. Such disasters leave a sense of shock or disbelief. How could this have happened? What does it mean? Disasters can shake our belief in our government, our way of life, the future of our planet, or our belief in God. Some disasters are natural, such as floods, earthquakes, or droughts; some are man-made, such as war, terrorism, chemical disasters, oil spills, and nuclear meltdowns. Others are both: for example, the effects of pollution, deforestation, and global warming.

Types of disaster are widely variable, of course, and so are the ways that people recover from them. When a disaster strikes close to home, the people affected may be left with symptoms of post-traumatic stress disorder. Some of the more obvious difficulties that come with PTSD are anxiety, insecurity, overreactivity, nightmares, flashbacks, difficulty sleeping, and depression. However, there are also aspects of post-traumatic stress disorder that can be concealed and yet are still very painful—the defenses, suppression, and disconnection. Suppression is a way to push thoughts and feelings out of awareness. Although the person may avoid consciously thinking about the trauma, nevertheless the suppressed emotions seek other outlets, such as through physical symptoms or by sudden intense or violent outbursts. Disconnection, another defense, severs the meaningful connections between experiences, thoughts, feelings, or values.

One form of disconnection is called *dissociation* and involves a kind of disowning of one's experiences, thoughts, and feelings such that they no longer seem to be part of one's self. Suppression, disconnection, and dissociation represent the mind's last-ditch defenses against unbearable psychic pain. These defenses enable the person to keep functioning but at a great emotional cost. For example, they can result in a loss of cognitive and emotional flexibility, impaired relationships, anxiety, depression, self-destructive behaviors, substance abuse, emotional isolation, rage attacks, loss of meaning in life, loss of creativity, reduced ability to work, and physical pain and illness.

Prior to industrialization, most disasters were the result of wars or natural causes such as floods, fires, earthquakes, volcanic eruptions, or infectious epidemics. Unfortunately, because our habitats are now filled with synthetic substances, when a disaster occurs—for example, Hurricane Katrina, the September 11 World Trade Center attacks, the Exxon *Valdez* and Deepwater Horizon oil spills, or the nuclear disasters in Chernobyl and Japan—toxic substances are released into the environment, substances that can affect people and other living things for decades. First responders and area residents in a disaster area may suffer from direct skin contact with chemical toxins; even more frequently, they suffer from inhaling toxins that are released into the air. Consequently, many responders and survivors suffer from both emotional stress along with respiratory problems that include upper-airway disease, chronic cough, vocal cord dysfunction, difficulty speaking, lung infiltrates, and increased risk of cancer. Over time, after the toxins contaminate water, they may appear in crops, seafood, and livestock. Survivors therefore may have to cope not just with the immediate trauma, the loss of family and friends, the loss of a home or a job, and the impaired health that may follow a disaster, but also with uncertainty regarding possible long-term health consequences. During what is supposed to be the recovery period, the stress-response system cannot rest because the survivor cannot feel safe, even after the disaster.

A small number of studies using mind-body practices for mass disasters have been published, but more work needs to be done. It is extremely difficult to conduct scientific studies in the aftermath of a mass disaster. However, those studies that have been done show highly beneficial effects. In the following sections, we will describe breath practices that have been used to help people in their recovery from the 2001 World Trade Center terrorist attacks, the 2004 Southeast Asian tsunami, the 2010 earthquake in Haiti, the war and genocide in Rwanda, and the war and slavery in Sudan.

You will learn how these practices can be used not only for individual recovery from such mass disasters but also to improve disaster preparedness and community resiliency.

September 11 World Trade Center Attacks

Eight years after September 11, 2001, an estimated four hundred thousand people were said to be still suffering from the physical and psychological effects of the attacks on the World Trade Center. We acquired firsthand experience with these problems while working with a small nonprofit, Serving Those Who Serve (STWS), to provide holistic treatments for first responders, Ground Zero workers, and others affected by the World Trade Center attacks. One of the founders of STWS, Nehemiah Bar Yehuda, attended a breath workshop with us. In 2007, he and two other STWS founders, José Mestre and Marshall Saul Stackman, invited us to do a program for the September 11 community. During and after the workshop, participants experienced profound emotional relief and many felt better physically. As a result, STWS began sponsoring regular Breath~Body~Mind workshops. Most of the people who attended our workshops had already been through years of standard psychiatric and medical treatments but were still ill. Several have offered to share their stories.

TWO-TIME ESCAPEE

Sonya was working in the World Trade Towers in 1993 and was evacuated from the building when terrorists detonated a truck bomb beneath the North Tower. After the attack, she developed post-traumatic stress disorder, for which she received psychotherapy. She managed to keep her job, but during the summer of 2001 she began having recurring nightmares of an impending disaster. She was working on the eightieth floor of one of the towers when terrorists attacked again in September 2001. This time, as she was trying to escape down the stairwell, she became too exhausted to keep going. Fortunately, two men supported her all the way down to the basement. They emerged in pitch darkness not knowing which way to go. Only the light of a policeman's flashlight in the distance guided them out to the street and safety before the entire structure collapsed. After this harrowing escape, Sonya had severe PTSD with anxiety, nightmares, and constant distress. She tried conventional and alternative treatments, including some Resistance Breathing (*ujjayi*) with no improvement. In 2008, seven years after the disaster, she attended our Breath~Body~Mind workshop and participated in the study we were conducting. Not only did she report feeling much better, but her test scores showed concrete improvement in all measures of anxiety, PTSD, and depression immediately after completing the workshop.[5]

VOCAL CORD DYSFUNCTION

Mike was a firefighter with the New York City Fire Department when terrorists attacked the World Trade Center in September 2001. Along with his brotherhood of other firemen, he was part of the initial rescue at the site and then worked every day for over a year dealing with the wreckage at Ground Zero. As a result of exposure to toxins he developed persistent hoarseness and difficulty speaking. Although he was not the type to talk about his feelings, he also showed signs of post-traumatic stress disorder. For five years he was treated by clinic doctors and hospital specialists, all to no avail. He was told that he would have to adjust to being hoarse for the rest of his life. Not one to give up, he took one of our Breath~Body~Mind workshop. By the end, his hoarseness was gone. Working at Ground Zero where his mind was exposed to the horror of human body parts and his body was exposed to toxic chemicals, the trauma became lodged in his throat. Breathing, movement, and meditation practices broke the link between the trauma and his throat, restoring normal speech.

In order to evaluate the impact of the Breath~Body~Mind practice on people affected by the September 11 attacks, we decided to do a research study. Having worked with Dr. Katzman and Dr. Vermani on the GAD studies, we asked them to join us for two open pilot studies of

Breath~Body~Mind practitioners affected by the September 11 terrorist attacks. Both studies demonstrated that the program significantly relieved symptoms of PTSD, anxiety, and depression.[6] This program has been further simplified so that the basic practices can be taught and provide some relief in one session lasting just a few hours.

GROUND-GLASS LUNGS

Following the World Trade Center attacks, doctors began to see lung infiltrates on X-rays of survivors that looked like ground glass, a condition called *ground-glass opacity* or *ground-glass lungs*. There was no specific cure for this condition, which tended to persist for years along with respiratory symptoms such as chronic cough. Two of the participants in our Breath~Body~Mind workshops had been taking ayurvedic detoxifying herbs for over a year with limited improvement. After completing the workshop and practicing the breath techniques daily for two months, they reported that their X-rays showed that the ground-glass infiltrates were clearing. They had received no treatment other than the breathing and the herbs. Coherent Breathing opens alveoli and fine airways in lung areas that are usually "dead space." The increased opening of lungs may have enabled the lungs to clear out more of the toxins. Many people with respiratory problems report that during the first several weeks of practice, their sinuses may drain or they may cough up large amounts of sputum as their lungs clear.

Scientific Studies of Mind-Body Programs for Mass Disasters

The majority of studies on the psychological effects of mass disasters document only the occurrence of symptoms. Very few study the effects of treatment in the aftermath of a disaster because the area may have lost the infrastructure needed to support research, or the area may be inaccessible or dangerous. Here are some of the available studies.

Dr. Shirley Telles is the director of research at Patanjali Yogpeeth, originally founded by Ram Dev, in Haridwar, India. She is also the principal investigator at the Indian Council of Medical Research for Advanced Research in Yoga and Neurophysiology at the Swami Vivekananda Yoga Research Foundation in Bangalore, India. Dr. Telles and her team conducted a randomized study of the effects of a one-week yoga program of one-hour-a-day yoga practices with breathing for twenty-two survivors one month after the August 2008 flood in Bihar, India. The flood killed 250 people, destroyed more than 300,000 homes, and displaced three million people. In a highly populated area of very fertile land, more than 840,000 acres of crops were lost. Survivors who participated in the one-week yoga sessions showed a significant decrease in sadness, whereas subjects in the control group had an increase in anxiety. That this yoga program appeared to reduce feelings of sadness while preventing an increase in anxiety suggests more generally that mind-body practices could help prevent the development of anxiety disorders such as PTSD following disasters—a possibility that warrants further study.

2004 TSUNAMI IN SOUTHEAST ASIA

A controlled study of 183 survivors of the 2004 Indian Ocean tsunami compared an eight-hour group yoga-breath program, alone or followed by three to eight hours of individual trauma-reduction exposure sessions, with a wait-list control group. Refugees who scored fifty or above on the Post-traumatic Stress Checklist (PCL-17), meaning their PTSD symptoms were moderate to severe, were assigned by camps to one of three groups: (1) yoga-breath intervention; (2) yoga-breath intervention followed by trauma-reduction exposure therapy; or (3) a six-week wait-list. Measures of PTSD (based on the checklist) and depression based on the Beck Depression Inventory (BDI-21) were performed as a baseline when the study began and then again at six, twelve, and twenty-four weeks. The effect of treatment compared to control was highly significant at six weeks: mean scores on the PTSD checklist declined 42.52 points with the yoga-breath program; 39.22 points with the yoga-breath treatment plus the exposure therapy; and only 4.61 points in the control group. After six weeks, decreases of at least 60 percent in mean scores on the PTSD checklist and 90 percent on the depression measure occurred in the groups that were given breathing treatments either alone or followed by exposure sessions, but there was no change in the control group. Most of the improvement occurred within the first week. The benefits were maintained at twenty-four-week follow-up. This study showed that breath practices dramatically and rapidly reduced symptoms of PTSD and depression and that the effects were long-lasting.

2010 GULF OF MEXICO OIL SPILL

The people of coastal Texas, Louisiana, Mississippi, Alabama, and Florida were threatened with toxins from the 2010 Deepwater Horizon oil spill in the Gulf of Mexico, along with devastation to wildlife populations, loss of income from fishing and tourism, and unknown health consequences. This disaster stuck economically depressed areas where the people had not yet recovered from a bruising series of hurricanes and floods. The Mississippi Department of Mental Health issued grants funded by the British Petroleum (BP) company and targeted at creating innovative approaches to address the ongoing high level of human stress associated with the oil spill. We were fortunate to obtain one of these grants in 2011. This made it possible for us to train health-care workers and other service providers such as relief volunteers, teachers, and clergy in Breath~Body~Mind techniques that they could use in their work with people affected by the BP oil spill.

Caregivers who live in disaster areas have the double burden of helping their clients cope with the trauma while at the same time dealing with their own trauma-related losses and symptoms. This kind of caregiver stress can lead to burnout, a condition of exhaustion in which the person feels depressed, helpless, defeated, and stressed. Burnout from stress or overwork can occur in any job, but people working in areas affected by disasters are even more susceptible. The adrenaline rush that energizes people to deal with a disaster cannot last. Eventually, exhaustion sets in. The person must keep working despite feeling that all their efforts are not enough. This can lead to poor job performance, irritability, family problems, and substance abuse.

Out of 170 people who participated in the three-day Breath~Body~Mind trainings funded by the grant, ninety attendees volunteered to participate in a research study. Dr. Chris Streeter, associate professor of psychiatry at Boston University Medical School, administered tests before the training, immediately after the training, and then five weeks later to determine its effects. Streeter's measurements, recorded on a "Perceived Stress Scale," showed high levels of stress before the training and very significant improvements following the training. Another measurement, the "Exercise Induced Feeling Inventory," documented highly significant improvements in engagement, revitalization, tranquility, and energy.

Many of the counselors and therapists who completed the training have reported excellent results when they teach the practices to their clients. Some of these practitioners work with homeless families and people whose jobs vanished because of the environmental disaster. It was rewarding for them to discover that despite living in a desperate situation, many of their clients found relief from the movement and breathing practices.

Mass Disasters in Countries with Few Resources

Mass disasters overwhelm health-care resources even in developed countries such as the United States and Japan. The situation is even more critical in countries lacking such resources, where there may be little or no remaining infrastructure and few if any professional health care providers.[7]

HAITI EARTHQUAKE OF 2010
The situation following the 2010 earthquake in Haiti provided the impetus for us to develop a shorter set of breathwork practices that could be taught

in one session anywhere, anytime, with no technology. Our work in this instance began with a phone call from Gretchen Wallace, a breathwork trainer and president of Global Grassroots, one week after the earthquake devastated Haiti. Gretchen was very experienced in doing therapeutic breathwork one-on-one with her clients but not in teaching breathwork to large groups. She asked us to suggest a simple set of practices that could be quickly taught to earthquake survivors, because she was about to fly to Haiti as a volunteer. Choosing elements of our usual two-day program, we suggested three simple qigong movements and the basic breath practices. The following weekend a group of yoga teachers joined us for a quick training. One of them, Barbara Johnson, an integrative breathwork practitioner, accompanied Gretchen to Haiti and kept a journal.

Two weeks after the earthquake, Gretchen met with a group of fifty Haitian women with symptoms of acute post-traumatic stress disorder, who were living in the crumbled ruins of a slum along the Bourdon Valley, just south of Port-au-Prince. Working through AMURTEL (Ananda Marga Universal Relief Team — Ladies), an international NGO (nongovernmental organization) that had been operating an orphanage in the community for eight years, Gretchen was introduced to a group of village women. In one evening, she discussed the effects of trauma and taught the women the qigong movements, "Ha" breath, belly breathing, and Coherent Breathing. The women responded immediately with feelings of relaxation, calmness, and relief of physical discomforts.

Gretchen recalled, "They brought one woman to sit in front of me. I guessed she was in her fifties or sixties. Her eyes were glazed over. She looked completely numb and could not even look me in the eye. Instead, I held her rough hands and breathed again with her, overexaggerating the sound of my breath so that she might hear me. She slowly began to mirror my pace, at five breaths per minute. We breathed like this together for a few more minutes and I invited others to join. A second short breathing session followed. When we finished, the woman nodded and smiled."
When Gretchen returned to Haiti two weeks later, the group had contin-

ued to meet weekly to practice on their own, and they had brought more women to learn and practice with them.

Barbara Johnson's journal entries describe what happened:

March 7, 2010:

Later in the afternoon, we followed the *didis* (nuns) and AMURTEL staffers by car to Citron, an IDP (internationally displaced persons) camp up the valley. The *didis* had arranged for us to do our program with the women of the camp. We arrived at a new (since the quake) community of about one hundred huts made from sheet metal, plywood, and tarps. The residents' former homes were visible across the valley, crumbled into landslides.

We brought huge UN tarps to spread in a clearing in the midst of the huts where a big crowd was gathering. Women and girls immediately began seating themselves, and soon there were one hundred or more on the tarps, with more standing off to the sides with as many men and boys. It appeared to be a barely manageable crowd. We were packed onto those tarps, surrounded by a din of Creole. Gretchen thanked the women for coming, acknowledged their difficulties, and said we hoped to help them with a practice that had helped others in similar circumstances. Then she described our bodies' response to a traumatic experience: sleeplessness, nightmares, numbness, vigilance, worry, trouble breathing, nervousness, digestive troubles, back pain, etc. She asked the group if any had experienced these things. Most of the women nodded and many affirmed her list of symptoms. They began talking about how knowing this was such a relief because they had thought that the symptoms meant that they were going crazy.

We told them we would be doing some movement and breathing together. We asked them to stand up, and we demonstrated the shaking movement, arms hanging like ropes. Many were shy, laughing, holding back, but most of them got going. The men and boys were hooting. Next we did "Ha" Breath . . . BIG hit. One tiny old lady really got into it. The guys did it, too. Next, I lay down in the center of the group and demonstrated belly breathing. We asked them to lie down and begin to breathe with one hand on their belly and one on their chest, so they could feel themselves fill their lower breathing space. Gretchen rang a tiny bell into the microphone to time the breathing.

They were all stretched out, taking up every inch of those tarps, the young girls piled up like puppies. The group energy felt sky-high when we began, but immediately calmed down. It was amazing how they settled. I asked them to relax their jaws, eyes, hands, and feet; just breathe, be still, pay attention to the breath. We only went for five to seven minutes, then did a body scan, and asked them to feel how much calmer the group was, all because each of them was a little calmer. We told them they could do this when they feel upset or anxious, or if they want to sleep. We had them sit up and asked how they felt. They felt better, calmer, and had less pain. They were delighted to have the opportunity to come together and learn techniques to feel better. Gretchen told them that if they do this morning and evening, they will feel better and better and breathe easier. We ended standing, the group singing and swaying. Yet, I saw one hard face that seemed unmoved—I wondered then and now what she had been through and how she felt about all this.

COHERENT BREATHING IN RWANDA

Survivors of genocide in countries like Sudan and Rwanda have been victims or witnesses of atrocities and suffering including murder, rape, torture, starvation, HIV infection, and severe deprivation. Such individuals often function by suppression of feelings and memories. When these are triggered, they may lose control of their minds and their reactions.

In Rwanda every April there is an annual commemoration of the 1994 genocide, which killed nearly one million people in one hundred days. Gretchen Wallace recalled, "My first visit to Rwanda was in 2006 during the twelfth anniversary of their genocide. I found myself one of only three white Westerners surrounded by nearly seventy-five hundred mourners who had just exhumed the bodies of their family members from mass graves for a proper burial. The remains of up to thirty people occupied each coffin. A parade of pickup trucks led the way carrying nearly two hundred caskets neatly draped with purple crosses soaked with tears from family members. Our destination was the Kigali Memorial Centre, surrounded by underground tombs where fifty thousand massacred Tutsi rested nine coffins deep.

"As the survivors assembled, the quiet distress that must permeate every day for people living side-by-side with their family's murderers began to flood the senses. Mourners crowded together under tents. Suddenly a woman screamed. Trauma workers in red first-aid vests dove into the crowd to reach the woman and lead her away arm-in-arm, dragging her feet, sobbing and screaming. The fragile facade crumbled and the collective wound began to spew up the grief, anger, and sadness as survivors unwillingly relived or uncontrollably released their pain. I caught a glimpse of a back room full of women who had been extracted from the crowd. Most sat slumped against the wall. Attendees fanned them or sang softly while the women sobbed. Others slept. I asked a staff person what would happen tomorrow to support these women. 'Nothing,' was the answer. 'They go back to normal life, like everyone else.'"

Global Grassroots' Academy for Conscious Change in Rwanda has incorporated breathwork, yoga, meditation, mindfulness, and other consciousness practices into its eighteen-month social entrepreneurship program for women in Rwanda since the program's founding there in 2006. Gretchen finds that even now, seventeen years after the genocide, mind-body techniques, especially the core Breath~Body~Mind practice, can provide psychological healing that is essential for personal transformation as well as social change. Years after their initial training, the women continue to utilize these practices to support their recovery and to manage stress from their life of poverty.

Ellen Ratner, the host on the Talk Radio News Service who is experienced in mental health care, attended many of our workshops and practiced breathwork regularly. She had been working with Dr. Luka Deng in a rural clinic in South Sudan, about thirty miles from Darfur, with genocide survivors and with women and children recently rescued from years of slavery in North Sudan. Believing that breath practices would relieve their symptoms of depression and trauma, she invited us to participate in helping them by creating a breathwork practice that she could teach; she pointed out that there were no mental health treatments or services in that area and that training in breathwork would be the only psychological intervention they were likely to receive. Assuming that these survivors had complex trauma and that some of them probably needed to use suppression (blocking out their thoughts and feelings about the traumas), we did not want to teach any practices that might trigger trauma memories. Therefore, we suggested a few simple qigong movements and Coherent Breathing, followed by rest. Ellen returned from Sudan reporting very positive responses to the program; she saw improvements in levels of worry, fear, jumpiness, mood, and physical pain. One of the village matrons had taken over the task of ringing a chime bowl to lead the breathing. Ellen asked us to evaluate the effectiveness of the program with her next group of survivors.

When Dr. Luka Deng and Ellen decided to evaluate the effects of the breathwork program, we sent two psychological scales to assess levels of depression and post-traumatic stress disorder. These tests were given to nineteen Sudanese women who were survivors of war and genocide traumas. Five days a week the women came to the clinic, where the staff led them in three qigong movements and twenty minutes of Coherent Breathing. The tests of mood and PTSD were repeated after six and eighteen weeks. The results after eighteen weeks of practice showed a 66 percent improvement in mood scores and a 71 percent improvement in PTSD symptom scores. While this was not a controlled study, it suggested that even in extremely traumatized disaster survivors, a simple twenty-minute practice of movement and breathing could significantly relieve symptoms of depression and PTSD.[8]

In July 2011, Ellen Ratner and Dr. Brown traveled to Dr. Luka Deng's clinic during the week prior to South Sudan's declaration of independence from the North; the intent was to provide stress and trauma relief using Breath~Body~Mind practices for six hundred recently liberated slaves, mostly women and children. The former slaves walked for seven days with bare feet or flip-flops through jungle and desert in extreme heat to reach the clinic in South Sudan before returning to their home villages.

Working through a translator, Dr. Brown led the first group of two hundred former slaves in simple qigong movements and breathing practices. Within about fifteen minutes, the grim, frozen faces with vacant stares transformed, as the Sudanese began smiling, laughing, breathing, and eventually dancing. It was as though they could finally unfreeze their emotions and feel some joy and hope. Two days later he saw the same response as he taught a group of four hundred women and children. He also worked with eighteen severely disabled polio victims, who felt that the gentle movement and breathing practices would increase their strength, mobility, and independence.

Dr. Brown also worked with the twenty women, former slaves, who had learned the practices from Ellen Ratner and who had been practicing Coherent Breathing for six to twelve months. He led them into more advanced techniques, inducing deep and powerful stress release. Afterward, the women expressed their intention to travel to other villages where they would teach the practices to more women and children.

Independence was declared at the end of the week. For the Sudanese, their flag is a very important symbol of independence. They used crayons to create flags on pieces of paper and taped these to sticks. Despite the years of misery and deprivation, every man, woman, and child held up their flags with the hope of a better future for their country.

Caregiver Stress and Secondary Trauma

When caregivers are exposed to extreme suffering, they may experience adverse effects called "caregiver stress," "secondary (or vicarious) trauma," and "burnout." Whether you are taking care of a relative who is ill, or working in a hospital emergency room, or volunteering to help victims in a mass disaster, it is crucial to know your limits, to prepare yourself, to practice self-care techniques, and to participate in group support with coworkers. When caregivers become impaired by overwhelming stress, anxiety, exhaustion, frustration, or fear, they are not able to effectively help others. This becomes even more relevant for community providers who are caught in the disaster themselves and whose families are under severe stress. Caregivers need to use techniques to manage their own stress, anxiety, depression, anger, and sense of helplessness.

Barbara Johnson wrote in her Haiti journal on March 9, 2010, "This day we gave the program to a group of volunteers assembled by Kelly at the Haiti Relief Coalition, with the recognition that they, too, were stressed without much relief. We were in an airy house and we had a sound system for the 'Two Bells' [track 3 on the *Respire-1* CD]. They expressed physical feelings that we identified as releasing trauma. One overwhelmed mother of a toddler fell asleep. We had them breathe for ten minutes, finished with a Native American chant which sounded lovely. They all noticed the difference in the way they felt. Kelly told us she'd not been so relaxed since she arrived in Haiti."

Sustainability

Dr. James Gordon, medical director of the Center for Mind-Body Medicine in Washington, D.C., has organized multicomponent programs for relief of post-traumatic stress disorder in postwar Kosovo, Gaza, Palestine, and Israel, as well as for American soldiers and veterans. Dr. Gordon and colleagues conducted a randomized wait-list controlled study of eighty-two adolescents with PTSD in Suhareka, Kosovo. Classroom schoolteachers, supervised by psychiatrists and psychologists, provided the twelve-session mind-body skills program. Students had significantly lower PTSD symptom scores following the mind-body program compared with those in the wait-list control group and the improvements were maintained at a three-month follow-up.[9] Dr. Gordon's programs train people in each community to continue the work, while his staff provides periodic supervision.

As part of the Center for Mind-Body Medicine's Global Trauma Relief program, Dr. Gordon's approach is to give people tools for helping themselves. This means that the local people must be trained to do the work. His programs teach the local trainers about self-care and how to set up support networks. For example, in Gaza, his team trained 240 local providers who subsequently delivered programs to twenty-five thousand people. The twelve-week program can include between nine to twelve techniques from the following list: slow breathing, meditation, biofeedback, movement, guided imagery, autogenic training, genograms and drawings, shaking and dancing, and simple written exercises. Programs can be adapted to the needs of each culture. (More information is available at the center's Web site, www.cmbm.org.)

Advantages of Mind-Body Practices for Disaster Relief

Mind-body practices have been used as primary methods for healing in traditional cultures for thousands of years; in modern times they have also been used by nonprofit and religious organizations to provide emotional relief in countries afflicted by disaster. Mind-body programs for relief of immediate and long-term effects of mass disasters offer the following advantages:

1. Mind-body practices can be conducted in groups, such that a small number of teachers can serve large numbers of disaster survivors.
2. Appropriate programs may provide rapid relief.

3. Programs can be tailored to different cultures so that they are easily understood and accepted.
4. They require no equipment, no electricity, no specific spaces, and no supplies.
5. They are lower cost because they require fewer professionals and minimal equipment. Once the members of the local community are trained to provide the intervention, mind-body programs become even more cost-effective and accessible, as local providers are better able to reach outlying areas.
6. Programs with simple techniques are easy to learn and easy to teach community leaders, who sustain and multiply the benefits.
7. Well-designed programs are highly sustainable. The psychological effects of mass disasters can last for years, even decades, and mind-body programs can continue to be a sustainable resource within communities for the ongoing long-term treatment and support needed following mass disasters.

Inoculate against the Effects of Trauma

More and more people and governments are realizing the need for disaster preparedness. We usually think that being prepared means having a flashlight, radio, first-aid kit, escape plan, and enough food and fresh water for several weeks. Public education and common sense have convinced most people to prepare for physical survival in the event of a disaster. But another important element in disaster preparedness is having a set of tools for emotional survival. During and immediately after a disaster, rescue and physical safety have top priority. The stress response is in high gear, providing the adrenaline needed for immediate survival. However, during the long-term recovery phase after a disaster, the cleanup and reconstruction, as people realize their losses, and as their stress-response systems become exhausted, what happens to the emotional trauma they carry? As thousands have discovered, it is easier to rebuild a flattened house than to repair shattered nerves.

History has shown repeatedly that treatments to ameliorate the psychological consequences of mass disasters are often ineffective or unavailable after the event. We may not know exactly when or where the next disaster will occur, but we know that more disasters are inevitable. It would be far more effective to inoculate against trauma so that when a disaster strikes, the survivors will already know how to preserve mental health and resilience for themselves, their families, and their neighbors.

Along these lines, programs are being developed that focus on creating "community resiliency." For example, the Trauma Resolution Center of Miami offers stress resiliency workshops for professionals and the general public. The center's founder, Teresa Descilo, points out that "besides the possibility of natural disasters, very few people go through life without being impacted by some crushing event. We work with thousands of victims of trauma every year. In order to prevent compassion fatigue and maintain stress resilience, my staff engages in regular mind-body practices that include breathwork, meditation, yoga, qigong, and sound bowls. We share these techniques with other community agencies. These practices can be used in the workplace, faith community, and at home. After the severe hurricane season of 2005, the Children's Trust provided funding for our 'Relax Miami' program. When the Red Cross funded our community-wide service in 2008, we named it 'Building Community Resiliency.'"

Considering the unpredictability of many disasters, preventive measures could reduce the burden of psychological consequences. Training in simple mind-body practices could provide trauma inoculation. Community resiliency training would empower people to reduce anxiety, difficulty sleeping, fatigue, and physical disorders caused by experiencing a mass disaster in situations where there may be no mental health care providers or medications, where there may be no help of any kind for days, weeks, or even months.

In conclusion, evidence from research and the experience of those who work with disaster survivors indicate that mind-body interventions are feasible and beneficial during and after disasters. Mind-body practices offer inexpensive, effective treatment for PTSD and wellness support for survivors of war and natural disasters, which is critical to both personal healing and the reconstruction processes. Gretchen Wallace observed that when treatment for PTSD is available, survivors are better able to heal from medical injury. They are also able to attend more resourcefully and resiliently to needs not addressed by relief aid, which may be limited or delayed. Psychological trauma relief also helps survivors forge bonds within the community to solve problems collectively rather than resorting to violence for self-preservation.[10] Furthermore, where the mental health infrastructure is destroyed by disaster, simple, cost-effective solutions that are easily learned, sustained, and taught across multiple language and cultural barriers—especially those that do not require a long-term client-practitioner therapeutic relationship—will have the broadest impact.

How to Use Breath Practices in Sickness and in Health

For healthy people who have mild to moderate stress, twenty minutes of Total Breath practice once a day is usually sufficient. However, during periods of greater stress, it helps to practice twice a day. Once you learn how to do Coherent Breathing, you will notice feeling more relaxed during and immediately after you practice. As you continue to practice, the benefits will last longer and you will discover how easy it is to shift into breathing at five breaths per minute anytime during the day without skipping a beat when you feel stressed.

For people with anxiety or depression, we recommend twenty minutes twice a day. Total Breath is best done in the morning. Because some people find Breath Moving to be activating, we recommend simple Coherent Breathing or Coherent Breathing plus Resistance Breathing at night to facilitate sleep. During the day, Coherent Breathing, Resistance Breathing, and Breath Moving can be used as often as necessary to prevent or minimize anxiety. After practicing daily for three months, Coherent Breathing with or without Resistance Breathing can be done on and off all day long except during physical exertion. The focused practice with eyes closed should continue to be done once or twice a day as needed.

Stress and physical illness are usually intertwined. Having a medical problem and undergoing tests or procedures can be highly stressful, even traumatic. Feeling ill or being in pain is stressful and may set off anxieties about health and the future. Also, stress can exacerbate medical problems such as ulcers, high blood pressure, and heart disease. For stress that is the result of dealing with medical illness, as well as for stress-related medical illnesses, twenty minutes of breathwork twice daily plus on and off breath practice during the day can be very helpful. Furthermore, fear intensifies the experience of pain, so in many cases, by alleviating anxiety, it is possible to reduce the level of pain related to illness by more than half. In more general terms, when being ill leads to feelings of helplessness, using breath practices in the ways described above can empower a person to control anxiety and reduce pain—that is, to feel less helpless.

Anyone who wishes to optimize physical and mental health can benefit from doing these breath practices, including doing the focused twenty-minute practice and also the on-and-off practice while engaged in daily activities.

5

Good Vibrations

"Ha" Breath, Breath Counts, the Total Practice, Vibration Breathing with Om *and* Song, Kong, Tong, Dong

> In the beginning was the Word and the Word was with God and the Word was God.
>
> Amen (Aum)
>
> —Book of John 1.1

> Om is the primordial throb of the universe. It is the sound form of Atma (Consciousness).
>
> —Maitri Upanishad *(c. 800–400 B.C.E.)*

Now that you are familiar with the Total Practice of movement, breathing, and meditation, it is time to introduce you to other healing breath techniques. First you will learn the activating, energizing "Ha" Breath and the use of Breath Counts. These will be followed by an exploration of two forms of Vibration Breathing: the universal *om (aum)* and the chant *"song, kong, tong, dong"* taught by the qigong master Robert Peng.

Awaken Your System with "Ha" Breath

Stimulating breath practices help increase mental alertness. When the mind is fuzzy or disorganized, "Ha" Breath will bring it into focus. We strongly advise that "Ha" Breath and other stimulating forms of breathing only be done for brief periods of time, no more than five minutes. For most people two to five minutes is all that is needed. However, it can be done two or three times throughout the day.

"Ha" breathing has been practiced for thousands of years by millions of people in different lands. For most people, it is a safe, invigorating practice, but there are some contraindications. Because this is a forceful, stimulating practice, "Ha" breathing should not be done by people who have uncontrolled hypertension, seizure disorder, pregnancy, recent surgery, aneurysm, hernia, or bipolar disorder. The internal pressure generated by forceful exhalation can transiently elevate blood pressure. Rapid forceful breathing may trigger a seizure in people with epilepsy. If you have had recent surgery, an aneurysm, or a hernia, the last thing you need is increased internal pressure. In people with bipolar disorder, any stimulating practice can cause mood changes with euphoria, agitation, irritability, or other manic symptoms.

There are many ways to do "Ha" breathing. The instructions in the box below describe an approach that most people find to be simple and effective. Track 5 leads you through "Ha" Breath.

"Ha" Breath

- Stand up straight, with your elbows bent, palms pointed upward, fingers curved into loose fists.
- Inhale, breathing deeply through your nose while retracting your elbows behind your back, palms facing upward, hands in loose fists.
- Exhaling sharply, make the sound, "Ha!" loudly, while you extend your arms and throw your hands forward, letting your palms turn

downward. Thrust your hands forward as though you are fling-
ing water off the tips of your fingers. As you fling your hands forward, let go of any tension in your hands and fingers.
- Inhale deeply, palms pointed upward, bending your elbows and
drawing them back, hands in loose fists.
- Exhale sharply with the "Ha" sound, repeating the same arm
movements.
- This should be done briskly, approximately one breath per second
—that is, you should breathe both in and out during one second.
- "Ha" breath can be done for fifteen repetitions (fifteen seconds)
or for up to three minutes continuously, depending on your physical capacity and on how much is needed to activate your system.

When to Use "Ha" Breath

"Ha" Breath is great for waking up in the morning or for when you're feeling tired during the day. When you need to study or do intellectual work
for a prolonged period of time and find that your mind is getting fuzzy or
unfocused, a few minutes of "Ha" breathing will get you back on track.
For the best effects, don't hold back. Sing out loud and strong when you let
loose with your "Ha!"

Contraindications to "Ha" Breathing

Remember, "Ha" breathing should not be done by people who have
uncontrolled hypertension, seizure disorder, pregnancy, recent surgery,
aneurysm, hernia, or bipolar disorder.

Attention Deficit Hyperactivity Disorder

Although people with attention deficit hyperactivity disorder (ADHD) may
appear to be overactivated, in fact parts of the brain responsible for focusing attention and for inhibiting inappropriate behavior are underactive.

"Ha" Breath can help to activate those "sleepy" parts of the brain to improve attention and behavioral control in people with ADHD or attention deficit disorder (ADD). Students with ADHD struggle with homework because they are not able to focus or organize their thoughts enough to complete assignments. Fear of failing at school creates secondary anxiety, and this anxiety further impairs cognitive performance. Breath practices such as "Ha" Breath followed by movement and breath counting (see below) can be particularly helpful. The "Ha" Breath activates attention, while breath counting and Coherent Breathing reduce anxiety and further enhance mental focus. Since people with ADHD tend to feel restless, they may be more comfortable doing breath practices with movements. The movements help to neutralize their physical agitation. The following vignette illustrates how to help a child with attentional problems using breath practices.

Although Charlie was an intelligent boy, in fourth grade he began having serious problems in school. As the work required more concentration, his ADHD became more of a liability. His grades fell from As to Cs and were heading further down. Realizing that Charlie was becoming frustrated and anxious, his parents brought him to Dr. Brown for help. First, he was taught the "Ha" Breath. Since children are usually told to be quiet, Charlie really enjoyed shouting "Ha!" as loud as he could. Next, he taught Charlie and his mother Coherent Breathing at six breaths per minute, so that mother and son could practice every day together at home. Charlie used "Ha" Breath to keep his mind alert when he noticed himself zoning out while doing homework. Coherent Breathing helped him to calm down, focus his mind, and feel more in control. He learned to use Coherent Breathing before sitting down to do homework and in preparation for tests at school. Charlie then began "experimenting" with his new skill. He found that doing breath practices before playing soccer improved his game by making him less distracted and better able to follow whatever was happening in the game. Like many people with ADHD, Charlie also tended to have trouble falling asleep. Using the "Two Bells" track on the *Respire-1* CD to pace Coherent Breathing made it much easier for him to fall asleep.

Breath Counts

"Ha" Breath is done so rapidly that it does not require counting. We use a CD to pace the breath while learning Coherent Breathing. This assures that the breathing is done at the desired rate. It also enhances relaxation by freeing the mind from the demands of counting. However, silently counting to time your own breath cycles also produces desirable effects. There are myriad ways to use counting in breath practices. Each cycle of breath has four potential phases: the in-breath, a pause, the out-breath, and another pause. The duration of each phase can be altered by counting. Depending on the relative length of each phase, different physiological effects are achieved. For example, when the out-breath is longer than the in-breath, there is greater stimulation of the parasympathetic system and the effect is mentally calming and physically relaxing. In the boxes below, we teach you a Breath Count that is widely used in yoga and qigong: 4-4-6-2. This means that you slowly count to four while breathing in, slowly count to four while pausing your breath, slowly count to six while letting your breath out, and slowly count to two while pausing your breath. This count is particularly effective when combined with movements, and it will enhance the physical and emotional benefits of movement practices.

Breath Counting with 4-4-6-2 in a Standing Position

- Stand with your feet shoulder-width apart. Straighten your head and relax your knees.
- Close your eyes and your mouth. Breathe in and out gently and slowly through your nose.
- Breathing in and filling your lungs, count slowly and silently: Breathe in . . . 2 . . . 3 . . . 4 . . .
- Pause and hold your breath as you slowly and silently count: Hold . . . 2 . . . 3 . . . 4 . . .

- Breathing out, count slowly and silently: Breathe out . . .
  2 . . . 3 . . . 4 . . . 5 . . . 6 . . .
- Pause and hold your breath as you slowly and silently count:
  Hold *. . . 2 . . .*
- Breathing in and filling your lungs, count slowly and silently:
  Breathe in *. . . 2 . . . 3 . . . 4 . . .*
- Hold your breath as you slowly and silently count: Hold *. . .*
  2 . . . 3 . . . 4 . . .
- Breathing out, slowly and silently count: Breathe out *. . .*
  2 . . . 3 . . . 4 . . . 5 . . . 6 . . .
- Hold your breath as you slowly count: Hold *. . . 2 . . .*
- Repeat this 4-4-6-2 breathing exercise for about five minutes.

Breath Counting 4-4-6-2 with Movement

This works particularly well for movements that involve stretching a muscle or tendon and holding the stretch. Breathing with the 4-4-6-2 count helps to relax the muscles, and the more the muscles relax, the more they can stretch. Also, some people forget to breathe while stretching. Breath counting assures a deep in-breath while the muscle and tendons are being stretched. Moreover, if you breathe in for four counts and hold for four counts, you will find that you can stretch further. This will be especially evident when you stretch the muscles of your back and torso, because when you inhale deeply, your chest will expand further. The expansion of the chest further stretches the muscles of the back and torso.

Movement with 4-4-6-2 Breath

- Stand with your feet shoulder-width apart. Straighten your head and relax your knees. Keep your arms down at your sides.
- Close your eyes and your mouth. Breathe in and out gently and slowly through your nose.
- Begin to raise your arms straight out from your sides and bring

your palms together above your head. As your arms are rising, breathe in . . . 2 . . . 3 . . . 4 . . .

- When your hands clasp above your head, point your index fingers toward the sky, and hold your breath as you slowly and silently count: Hold . . . 2 . . . 3 . . . 4 . . .
- (If you are able to raise your heels off the floor while doing this, even better.)
- Release your hands and slowly bring your arms back down to your sides, as you breathe out slowly, counting: Breathe out . . . 2 . . . 3 . . . 4 . . . 5 . . . 6 . . .
- Rest as you hold your breath, slowly counting: Hold . . . 2 . . .

You can repeat this breath and movement sequence as many times as you wish and use the 4-4-6-2 count with the rest of your movement practices. For example, try it with the Child Pose, as described in the box below.

Child Pose with 4-4-6-2 Breath

- Bend your knees to fold your legs beneath you as you rest with head, chest, arms, knees, and lower legs on the floor. Turn your head to one side. Rest your arms straight beside you with palms facing upward. Inhale slowly, counting: Breathe in . . . 2 . . . 3 . . . 4 . . . Notice how much more the back and shoulder muscles are being stretched.
- Hold your breath as you slowly and silently count: Hold . . . 2 . . . 3 . . . 4 . . .
- Slowly exhale as you relax, counting: Breathe out . . . 2 . . . 3 . . . 4 . . . 5 . . . 6 . . .
- Maintain the Child Pose position as you hold your breath while slowly counting: Hold . . . 2 . . .
- Repeat four to eight times.
- Staying in the same position, extend your arms straight out in front of you and let them rest on the floor with palms downward.

Inhale slowly, counting: Breathe in . . . *2* . . . *3* . . . *4* . . . Notice how the back and shoulder muscles are being stretched.
- Hold your breath as you slowly and silently count: Hold . . . *2* . . . *3* . . . *4* . . .
- Slowly exhale as you relax, counting: Breathe out . . . *2* . . . *3* . . . *4* . . . *5* . . . *6* . . .
- Maintain the position as you hold your breath while slowly counting: Hold . . . *2* . . .
- Repeat four to eight times.

The 4-4-6-2 breathing practice is also excellent for balancing the nervous system, the mind, and the emotions. It can be used every day whenever you like. If you or someone you know has anger management problems, you will find that doing five minutes of 4-4-6-2 with the arm movements can reduce anger, increase self-control, and avert damaging behaviors.

Obstacles to Breath Counting

Breath counting is not a natural rhythm. It can feel awkward at first. However, most people find it worth learning even though it may take a little practice. Here are some of the challenges that can arise while learning 4-4-6-2 and how to deal with them.

Can't Wait for the Next Breath

Some people have trouble holding the in-breath for four counts. If you run into this obstacle, just hold your breath for as long as you can without straining, and keep practicing. You will be surprised at how quickly it becomes easier to hold it for the full four counts. This is because your baroreceptors, special breathing receptors, learn to wait longer before signaling to your brain that you need more air.

Puffer Fish

One of our new students was having trouble with breath counting because he would quickly inhale as much as he possibly could, overfilling his chest with air like a giant puffer fish. Then, when he couldn't hold it any longer, he would spew it out with a great grunt. All this sucking in and spewing out was exhausting and hardly relaxing. He had to learn to go easy during all breath phases and not to overfill his lungs. The holding of the breath should be like a pause and not like holding back a flood of air.

More Ways to Use 4-4-6-2

The 4-4-6-2 Breath Count has beneficial effects on the nervous system. Each breath form is taught for its own special healing purposes. Just as you use different exercises for different muscle groups, you gain more by using a variety of breathing practices that each has their own unique effects. We want your entire system to work at its best. Here are some additional ways to make the most of the 4-4-6-2 breath.

Maintaining Attention

Some people find it easier to keep focused when using the 4-4-6-2 count compared to Coherent Breathing. For those whose mind tends to wander, the act of counting helps maintain focus. If you find that counting 4-4-6-2 is easier and it keeps your mind from wandering, then use it for your movement practices before you begin the Coherent Breathing part.

Breath Counting to Quiet Negative Thoughts

When you have time, it is good to do breath counting with movements before you begin Coherent Breathing. If you are having negative or suicidal thoughts, you may be able to alleviate them by doing some stretches along with 4-4-6-2 breathing. Negative thoughts may include ruminating—that is, going over and over the same scenarios in you mind. Usually these are things people said that hurt or angered you, things you wish you had said in reply, things you wish you hadn't said, things you plan to say the next time you see the offending person, things you said or did that embarrassed you, things you worry about in the future, and so on. Some negative thoughts appear as fears, for instance, worrying that one of your children will get hit by a car or worrying that someone will attack you as you walk down a street. Doing the complete practice every day and using 4-4-6-2 breathing with movement can help to quiet those recurring worrying thoughts.

One of our colleagues was concerned about the problem of suicidal feelings among a group of veterans who were hospitalized under his care. The veterans did not actually want to kill themselves, but they could not stop thoughts of suicide from coming into their minds over and over again. Dr. Brown suggested that he teach them a qigong practice called the Four Gold Wheels that he had learned from Master Robert Peng (www.robert peng.com). To enhance the effects, they should also use 4-4-6-2 breathing while performing the qigong movements. Several weeks later he called to report that five minutes of 4-4-6-2 breathing with the movements was enough to stop the suicidal thoughts in the veterans he was treating. Scientific studies would be needed to delineate the neurophysiological mechanisms that could explain this response. We would hypothesize that the 4-4-6-2 breathing has several positive effects including activating the serotonin system, which is often underactive in depression. Although the effects of 4-4-6-2 breathing on serotonin levels have not been studied scientifically, we discovered that when our patients have withdrawal symptoms from discontinuation of antidepressants that affect serotonin activity—for example, drugs such as paroxetine (Paxil) and venlafaxine (Effexor)—doing 4-4-6-2 breathing stops the withdrawal symptoms.

Changing the pattern of breathing can have powerful and rapid effects on our thoughts and feelings. If you are experiencing unwanted negative thoughts or destructive impulses that keep coming back, you may be able to make them stop with 4-4-6-2 breathing, breathing with movement, or Coherent Breathing with Resistance and Breath Moving. Try them all at different times and see what works best for you.

Breathing and Good Vibrations

Resistance Breathing creates an ocean sound by tightening the back of the throat; likewise, singing and chanting come from a tightening of the vocal cords in a way that causes turbulence in the air that creates sound waves. We can think of singing and chanting as forms of Resistance Breathing; these activities also stimulate the vagal nerves through slowing of the respiratory rate and increasing pressure in the lungs. The soothing effects of chanting or singing slowly are partly a result of slowing the breath rate and partly a result of prolonging the out-breath, both of which are known to stimulate the parasympathetic nervous system, the relaxing, healing, feel-good part of the nervous system. But the soothing outcome of chanting and singing is even more complex than this explanation implies, as you will see as we explore the effects of vocal vibration.

Sounds are waveforms that have many effects, not only through the ears but throughout the entire body. Sound is transmitted through water, and the human body is 98 percent water. Sounds cause the body to vibrate inside. Imagine all of the internal organs of the body vibrating as you sing or chant. Sit comfortably. Just close your eyes and sing this single long sound: *a . . . a . . . a . . . a . . . a . . . a . . . a . . . a . . . h.* As you sing, pay close attention to feeling the vibrations that this type of vocalizing creates, first in your belly and chest, and then radiating to your throat, head, hands, and feet. With a little practice, you should be able to feel the vibrations all the way down to your feet. You are able to feel these vibrations because they trigger sensors that send information through the vagal nerves to the brain. Vibrations through singing and chanting are another means to activate the vagus nerves and different parts of the brain.

Yoga and qigong teach that certain sounds affect different organs or energy centers, where they have healing effects. We will start with the most well-known yoga sound, *om,* and then show you a qigong chant, *song, kong, dong, tong.*

The Universal *Om*

According to Eastern traditions, the universe originated as a sound that can still be heard: *om* (or *aum*). The notion that the universe began with a word, a sound, or a vibration is found in many ancient religious texts, including the Judeo-Christian Bible. Modern physics suggests that the universe is made up of particles and waves. Sounds are waves that can cause particles to vibrate. Conversely, the oscillation of particles can produce sound waves. In yoga, the chanting of *om* is believed to connect the self to the universe. See below for a discussion of what modern scientists are discovering about *om.* Track 7 teaches vibrational breathing.

- Take a slow deep breath in, and as you breathe out, sing one low note: *o . . . o . . . o . . . o . . . m . . . m . . . m . . .*
- There can be three parts to the sound: *a . . . o . . . m . . .* As you chant, prolong each of the three parts of the sound: *a . . . .a . . . a . . . o . . . o . . . o . . . m . . . m . . . m . . .*
- Close your eyes and repeat *a . . . o . . . m . . .* three times, drawing the sound out longer as you notice the place in your body where each sound creates the most intense vibrations. Keeping your eyes closed after you complete the three long *a . . . o . . . m . . .* chants, notice how you feel.

You may chant *om* with two sounds or *aum* with three sounds, whichever feels best to you. Variations of the Hindu *om* are found in many religions. For example, the Hebrew word for peace, *shalom,* has the *a* sound in the first syllable and the *om* sound in the second. The Arabic greeting *salaam* also means peace. Similarly, the word *amen* has the *a* and *m* sounds. If you prefer to use a sound or word from your own belief system, feel free to do so. Find a word that has an *o* or *a* sound followed by an *m* sound, such as *shalom* or *salaam* or *amen* or *home.* Using a word that has a special, hopeful, or loving meaning for you can help shift thoughts and feelings in a positive way.

The sound *om* is usually chanted on a low note rather than a high note. Try singing *om* on a higher note and then on a lower note. The vibrations from a high note tend to stay in the throat and head, whereas lower notes vibrate better throughout the body.

Many words with sacred meanings, including *om,* are used as mantras. Traditionally, a word is not a mantra unless it is given along with instruction in other aspects of yoga by a yoga master. The mantra, often combined with hand gestures called mudras, is used in many ways: for example, to focus the mind, enter altered states of consciousness, or achieve enlightenment. Today we use the word *mantra* rather loosely to mean a word or phrase repeated silently in the mind or chanted out loud, usually during meditation, to engender positive thoughts and feelings. In this sense, *om* is one of an infinite number of possible mantras. The fact that *om* has been given such importance by so many great masters of yoga and meditation throughout the ages shows that it has clearly stood the test of time.

What Does Modern Science Say about Om?

In 2011, Dr. Bangalore G. Kalyani, Dr. Bangalore N. Gangadhar, and colleagues at the National Institute of Mental Health and Neurosciences, Bangalore, India, used functional magnetic resonance imaging (fMRI) to study the effects of chanting *om* on brain areas. The study incorporated a basic understanding that one of the branches of the vagus nerve innervates the ear canal, that branches of the vagus nerve can be activated by vibration, and that information about vibrations travels from the vagus nerve to reach many areas of the brain. The researchers hypothesized that chanting *om* would cause vibrational stimulation around the ears and would activate the auricular branch of the vagus nerves leading to deactivation (quieting) of specific brain areas. We also believe that in addition to stimulating the auricular branch, chanting *om* causes vibrations throughout the body that activate other branches of the vagus nerve. In this study, healthy volunteers were taught to chant *om* as they underwent fMRI brain scans. Comparisons of the scans before and during *om* chanting showed significant deactivation of brain areas involved in emotion processing, particularly in the limbic system (the amygdala on the right side as well as the hippocampus, the parahippocampal gyrus, the orbitofrontal cortex, the anterior cingulate cortex, and the thalamus on both sides. This study contributes significant evidence for the potential effects of sound-induced vibrations on emotion regulation. The vagus nerves are activated by vibration sensations throughout the body, not just in the area of the ears. By changing the pitch of the sound, it is possible to move the epicenter of the vibrations to different locations in the body. In ancient healing systems such as yoga and qigong, sounds are used to stimulate, strengthen, and heal the mind and the body. New technologies such as brain-imaging techniques make it possible to study with increasing precision the effects of chants on brain functions. This may lead to advances in the use of mind-body practices—for example, chanting of sounds—in correcting imbalances in emotion regulation and other critical brain functions.

When and How to Use Om

Chanting *om* three times is a good way to begin your breathing practices at any given moment. Prolong the sound and become aware of the vibrations throughout your body as you chant. Chanting *om* is also a wonderful way to enter meditation. If you wish to add *om* to your Total Breath practice, it is best to chant it three times after completing the movement practice and right before starting Coherent Breathing. And finally, have you ever noticed that singing in a group of people is different from doing it alone? Chanting *om* with a group of people can also be a powerful experience.

Song, Kong, Tong, Dong: The Healing Qigong of Master Robert Peng

Qigong is a system of movements, sounds, and visualizations used to increase and circulate qi (or chi), the energy of life, and to clear away emotional and physical "blockages" that impede the free flow of energy throughout the body. Chanting creates vibrations that penetrate all cells and tissues. These vibrations are believed to restore normal functioning within tissues and organs. Western medicine uses the power of vibration primarily to accelerate healing in muscles. In comparison, Eastern mind-body practices put greater emphasis on healing internal organ systems.

Starting from childhood, Master Robert Peng was taught the art of healing qigong by the famous monk Xiao Yao (1889–1985) of the renowned Ch'an Buddhist monastery, Shaolin.[1] Vibrational sounds are crucial in Master Peng's therapeutic work. He teaches a healing chant that uses the sounds *song, kong, tong, dong*—in which *song* means to relax, *kong* opens divine energy, *tong* is to embody divine energy, and *dong* means to understand thoroughly, to be insightful, and to see clearly. Instructions for completing one basic round of the practice appear in the box below.

Basic *Song, Kong, Tong, Dong* Practice: One Round

- For this practice, you may sit in a chair or on the floor as long as you are comfortable and your spine is straight. Place your hands in your lap with both palms facing upward. Move one hand to partly overlap the other with both palms facing upward. Let the lower hand cradle the upper hand. Move your hands closer until the tips of your thumbs just touch one another.
- Sit comfortably with your spine straight, hands resting in your lap, with your palms upward and the tips of your thumbs touching one another.
- Relax your eyebrows and smile slightly.
- Move your thumbs slightly apart and then gently rejoin them.
- Take a deep slow breath in and as you breathe out slowly chant the long low note *s . . . o . . . n . . . g . . .*
- Take a deep slow breath in and as you breathe out slowly chant the long low note *k . . . o . . . n . . . g . . .*
- Take a deep slow breath in and as you breathe out slowly chant the long low note *t . . . o . . . n . . . g . . .*
- Take a deep slow breath in and as you breathe out slowly chant the long low note *d . . . o . . . n . . . g . . .*

As you sing each sound, notice where it vibrates inside your body. Master Peng recommends breathing nine rounds of *song, kong, tong, dong* and combining it with Breath Moving. This helps move energy throughout the body. You learned to use Breath Moving with Coherent Breathing and Resistance Breathing in chapter 2. In *song, kong, tong, dong*, the attention is focused on feeling internal vibrations moving between the head, the bottom of the pelvis in the area called the perineum, and the feet. The lists in the box below show how to match each sound with the movement of vibrations during the nine rounds. You will see that only rounds 1 and 9 direct vibrations to the perineum. Rounds 2 through 8 move the vibrations from the feet to the head and the head to the feet.

Song, Kong, Dong, Tong: Rounds 1–9

ROUND 1

- Begin by sitting comfortably with your spine straight, hands resting in your lap with both palms facing upward. Your lower hand should cradle your upper hand, with the tips of your thumbs barely touching one another.
- Relax your eyebrows and smile slightly.
- Move your thumbs slightly apart and then gently rejoin them.
- Take a deep slow breath in, and as you breathe out, slowly chanting the long low note *s . . . o . . . n . . . g . . .* , move the vibrations from perineum to head.
- Take a deep slow breath in, and as you breathe out, slowly chanting *k . . . o . . . n . . . g . . .* , move the vibrations from head to perineum.
- Take a deep slow breath in, and as you breathe out, slowly chanting *t . . . o . . . n . . . g . . .* , move the vibrations from perineum to head.
- Take a deep slow breath in, and as you breathe out. slowly chanting *d . . . o . . . n . . . g . . .* , move the vibrations from head to perineum.

ROUNDS 2–8	VIBRATION MOVEMENT
song	feet to head
kong	head to feet
tong	feet to head
dong	head to feet

ROUND 9	VIBRATION MOVEMENT
song	feet to head
kong	head to feet
tong	feet to head
dong	head to perineum

After you complete these nine rounds of *song, kong, tong, dong,* sit quietly with your eyes closed and become aware of whatever is happening inside. You may use this practice to calm down whenever you feel agitated, anxious, or upset.

How Moving Attention or Vibrations to Different Parts of the Body Might Work

While there are many religious and philosophical writings about the effects of attention and vibration, Western science has no proven answers to how they might work. Nevertheless, we do know that focusing attention enhances perception and has significant effects on how we experience sensations, including having an effect on how the mind interprets and responds to sensory information. For example, focusing attention can be used to induce a hypnotic state. When a hypnotist says "Focus all your attention on your right hand and feel it getting warmer," you feel the right hand get warmer than the left. Nothing has happened to the right hand, yet it feels warmer. The focusing of attention can change the way the mind perceives a part of the body.

Focusing attention on one part of the body activates the connections between that part of the body and the places where it is represented in the brain, in the somatosensory cortex of the parietal lobe. Sensory information from inside the body, such as vibratory sensation, is received by the interoceptive insular cortex, located in the Sylvian fissure between the temporal and frontal lobes. According to Dr. Bud Craig's theory of interoception, this input plays a role in what the insular cortext "tells" the regulatory centers for the nervous, cardiovascular, digestive, endocrine, immune, and other systems.[2] For instance, depending on the messages from the body, the insula could tell the emotion center in the amygdala to calm down instead of overreacting. Since the insula connects input from the body with emotion memory centers, there is also the potential to correct or change how we experience and feel about parts of our bodies. In chapter 6, you will find an example of how breath practices corrected the way an abuse survivor experienced her body. We can also use breathing combined with a special kind of meditation called "Open Focus," developed by one of the pioneers of brain biofeedback, Dr. Les Fehmi, to change the way we experience pain: to make it tolerable or to eliminate it. If you are suffering from chronic pain, you can learn more about the Open Focus method at www.openfocus.com. Dr. Fehmi's books *The Open-Focus Brain* and *Dissolving Pain*, along with his CD sets for teaching Open Focus meditation, are available for purchase at his Web site, OpenFocus.com.

Regardless of where you are emotionally, spiritually, and physically, concentrated vibrations through chanting and visualization will help you move to a more joyful, peaceful, and satisfied state of mind. The more you work on your practices, the more connected you will feel with yourself, with others, and with the universe. You will begin to enhance your sense of balance in the world and within yourself through these breathing practices.

6

The True Self

Breathing Practices to Enhance Relationships, Love, and Bonding; Heal Trauma; and Promote Connectedness

> Thus breathing is the natural way to the heart. And so, collect your mind and conduct it by way of your breathing by which air passes to the heart and together with the inhaled air force it to descend into the heart and to stay there. And train it not to come out of there quickly; for at first this inner enclosure and restraint is very wearisome, but when it become accustomed to it, then on the contrary it does not like whirling without, because it is there filled with joy and happiness.
>
> —*Saint Nicephorus of Mount Athos*

Relationships are complex. We sometimes feel disconnected even from the people we love most. Many things, including stress, can affect our ability to enjoy feelings of love. Human beings are all born with the capacity to love—we are, in a sense, primed for bonding. We could not survive without it. We even have prosocial bonding hormones such as oxytocin, what has come to be known as "the cuddle hormone." Our brains have thousands of receptors just waiting to respond to oxytocin with warm, fuzzy feelings. During childbirth and breast-feeding, oxytocin is released, enhancing the maternal-infant bond. Hugging, stroking, making love, even having dinner with a group of friends—all of these activities release oxytocin.[1] So, with all this priming and hormonal activity, why is it so difficult to sustain love?

The capacity for love is an essential part of the original being within every human being. The original being is what we are when we begin life, with all of our natural feelings and potential for development intact, what some call our "true self." We begin life completely open, receptive, and ready for love. And then things happen to us, some good, others bad. The true self becomes covered with the layers of our experiences, attitudes we acquire, and defenses against hurts. When too many protective layers build up, we may lose sight of our true self. Sometimes our minds become so busy with the business of living, figuring things out, getting things we want, avoiding things we don't want, or making plans, that the intellect loses its connection with the heart. Breathing practices can help us find a path back to our true self, back to our heart.

For love to flourish, there must be trust and security. Negative experiences, especially early in life, can damage our capacity for trust and, thus, our capacity for love. As wonderful as love can be, it does make us vulnerable to being hurt. Abuse, neglect, abandonment, and betrayal can be so painful that the injured person may feel the need to build walls, layers of protection against deep emotional involvements and potentially devastating disappointments. The price can be an empty life of desperate loneliness, isolation, and loss of meaning. People who experience trauma can become emotionally disconnected from themselves as well as from other people. They may long to return to the way they used to feel, but be unable to find their way back. As we experienced in chapter 4, breath practices can calm the mind and emotions and relieve anxiety, including anxiety about trust and intimacy. Breaking the grip of past injuries and trauma, stimulating vagal pathways to the brain's emotion centers, and releasing more bonding hormones are some of the ways that breathwork can penetrate the layers of protection and restore the capacity to connect and to love.

Stressful Relationships

Family relationships can be stressful. Our approaches to adult relationships often stem from emotional patterns formed during childhood, when we see life through a child's eyes. They involve gut reactions that can be triggered in an instant by one look or a tone of voice, and they can be highly resistant to change. Sometimes breathing practices can open the mind to fresh insights about established relationships, as was the case with Roger, and with Tony and Jessica.

Brotherly Love

Roger always had problems with his older brother, Mark. Although he knew that if he were ever in real trouble, Mark would be there to help, he had many painful memories of Mark bullying and humiliating him. Even though they were grown and each had a family of their own, Mark still never seemed to tire of picking on his little brother. If Roger objected, Mark would raise his voice, yell, escalate the criticism in front of their wives and children, and stomp out of the house, ruining the evening. No matter how successful Roger was, no matter how hard he tried, Mark still managed to find fault with him. And whenever Mark criticized, Roger would choke with anger, unable to defend himself or fight back. On the one hand Roger wanted to maintain a close relationship between his family and Mark's, but on the other hand he dreaded every visit and the inevitable bruising criticism.

A friend convinced Mark to participate in one of our intensive breathing workshops. Doing rounds of breathing, movement, and meditation, Mark began to relax, open up, and let go. As he allowed the breath to take over, he felt himself become the breath, part of the flow of energy in the universe. This higher state of consciousness seemed to free him from the stresses that had cluttered his mind. He became more aware of his subtle internal feelings, more aware of other people's feelings and situations, and even more aware of feelings and situations from the past. He remembered his father holding a strap in his hand and reprimanding Mark: "You're the oldest, so you are responsible for all the others. You are responsible for whatever happened." With that memory, he understood his brother's behavior. If anything went wrong, Mark was held responsible. Mark was afraid that Roger would mess something up, and he would be blamed and strapped by their father. That fear was driving Mark's criticisms of Roger. Once Roger realized that Mark's blustering was covering a fear of being punished, his own fear of Mark's anger vanished. From that moment on, Roger was able to sit down with his brother and discuss the negative effects his criticisms were having on their relationship. He was surprised to discover that Mark was unaware that he had been so critical. He had a massive blind spot about his own behavior and what it was doing to Roger. He agreed to try not to criticize. Mark's blind spot is still there, but Roger is able to calmly remind his brother, thereby protecting himself and both families from the negative consequences of the past.

You Light Up My Life

When two people are close enough to form a loving bond and become a couple, they focus attention on one another as they share their hopes and aspirations. They often have some idealized and unrealistic ideas about one another that add to the glow of their love. As time goes on, as they go through real experiences together, some deeper truths about their differences and limitations become evident. People often have difficulty handling these disappointments, particularly when they cannot see that their initial expectations were somewhat unrealistic. If they are able to talk, share, understand, and support one another, they will become even closer. But all too often, people react to disappointments in their relationships with feelings of hurt, anger, and blame—negative feelings that shut out love. Sometimes this shutting out is a reaction to an event that creates stress or involves loss. The event could be a severe injury from an accident, a job loss, the death of a parent or child, or any other extreme stress to which one or both of the couple cannot adapt. Once the angry, negative, isolating reaction sets in for a person, it can be quite difficult to reverse. We saw this play out vividly in the interactions of one couple who came to our two-day breath workshop.

We did not know their history, and that they had temporarily lost their love for each other after a tragic accident, but Tony and Jessica did seem to be an odd couple when they came to our intensive breathing workshop. She was all smiles and warmth; he wore a stone-faced scowl. As the workshop progressed we noticed that from time to time Jessica's eyes would fill up with tears, which she quickly wiped away on her sleeve. There was no reaction from Tony. But finally, on the afternoon of the second day, Tony unexpectedly raised his hand. "I have something to say to my wife," he announced. A hush fell over the room as he turned to Jessica and said, "Three years ago you were in a car accident with our kids. You got Joey out of the car alive, but the baby died. In my heart I have been blaming you, blaming and hating you all this time. I know it wasn't your fault, but I was punishing you with silence, the way my mother used to punish me. I was wrong. I hope you will forgive me, because I really love you." Unable to speak, Jessica gazed into her husband's eyes.

What happened to Tony's anger, and how did he recover his loving feelings for Jessica? We were overjoyed to see their relationship restored, but we were also very interested in how the breath practices might have induced this change. This interest is not just idle curiosity. If we can understand more about how breathing helps people recover their emotional lives, it should be possible to develop these practices to be even more effective. We think that several processes are set in motion by breathwork and that the combined effects create the conditions for transformation. By applying a bit of Western science, we can gain further understanding of the multiple ways that breath practices may facilitate the healing of trauma, the recovery of the capacity for love, and the return to the true self.

Transformation Using
Western Scientific Paradigms

Trauma creates lasting impressions in the mind. These impressions may be stored in fixed formations, sometimes called schema,[2] that are very difficult to access, to open up, or to change by talk therapies. In this chapter we will present cases that illustrated our evolving neurophysiological model of how breath practices affect the mind. We discussed the role of breath practices in soothing, balancing, and strengthening the stress-response systems. This is important for trauma recovery, because until the stress-response system is functioning well, we cannot feel safe, and until we feel safe, we can neither access nor heal trauma formations. Now we will explore in greater detail these and other processes that enable us to experience love and intimacy.

In post-traumatic stress disorder the parasympathetic branch of the autonomic nervous system is underactive. Breath practices can activate the parasympathetic system so that it can play its part in calming the stress-response system and reducing emotional overreactivity. But the parasympathetic system is also importantly involved in the release of oxytocin, an essential hormone for bonding in humans and in many other species. (For example, researchers found that male prairie voles—a kind of prairie dog—are so extremely responsive to oxytocin that if a male vole was injected with that hormone, he would bond for life with the first female vole he saw).[3] Stimulating the parasympathetic system therefore not only makes us feel safer, but it may also create a greater propensity for bonding as it releases oxytocin.

We think it is entirely possible that during the two-day breath course, Tony's parasympathetic system was activated by the breathwork, enabling him to feel calmer, less stressed, and more open. Add to that a hefty surge of oxytocin, and he was more able to reestablish the emotional bond with his wife. The enhancement of bonding by oxytocin release is not the whole story but it probably accounts for a significant component of the transformations we saw in Tony and have seen in many other people.

Another change that occurs during breath practices is that different parts of the brain communicate better in solving problems. Dr. Stephen Larsen is a neurofeedback specialist and professor emeritus at SUNY New Paltz. In a 2008 study using electroencephalograms to record brain-wave patterns in people during breathing practices, Dr. Larsen and colleagues observed an increase in synchrony. Usually the electroencephalogram is rather chaotic looking as it registers brain waves arising from the electrical activity in many different parts of the brain. When people did breathing practices such as slow breathing with Resistance Breathing, as well as other breath forms, however, their electroencephalograms showed an increased synchrony, that is, the tendency for the peaks and valleys of the brain waves from diverse areas of the brain to line up in synchronous activity. In more experienced breathwork practitioners, all of the brain waves synchronized continuously, a phenomenon called "whole brain synchrony" by Dr. Les Fehmi,[4] a pioneer in neurofeedback and author of *The Open-Focus Brain* and *Dissolving Pain*. Increases in synchrony are associated with greater ability to solve complex problems.[5] Such changes may have contributed to Tony's sudden insight, his epiphany.

Tony had never been in psychotherapy. He was not accustomed to thinking about the connections between his present-day emotions and the experiences he had in childhood. For example, even as a young child, when Tony disappointed his mother, she withdrew and did not speak to him, sometimes for days, sometimes for weeks. This harsh punishment made him feel terribly bad about himself, and emotionally abandoned. During the breathing workshop, he put the pieces together by himself and realized that he was punishing his wife the way he was punished by his mother, and that those feelings and behaviors were not appropriate in his marital relationship. Like Tony, many people find that during and after practicing breathwork, they are better able to gain deep and lasting insights that help them to understand and resolve long-standing relationship problems.

Bonding Is Not Only between People: Connection and Disconnection

Bonding is the experience of creating a meaningful connection, and one can form a bond to many things beyond other people. Religious individuals feel a bond with God. Spirituality may include a sense of feeling connected with everyone and everyone on earth or even with the entire universe. Some people feel an intense patriotic bond to their country, to their ethnicity, to a peer group, or to other aspects of their identity. Such bonds enrich our sense of belonging and our sense of having a purpose, a meaning in our lives. Without these bonds, we can feel lost, alone, isolated, and without meaning.

Sometimes when a disaster strikes, people lose their belief in whatever was once most meaningful to them. Their world seems forever changed. Nothing makes sense. They feel disconnected. This uncomfortable sense of disconnection, one of the subtle but painful symptoms of post-traumatic stress disorder, can be very difficult to overcome. It is hard for a person to feel something when they have become disconnected not only from other people but also from their own sense of self. In many cases, these feelings persist for years and may not respond to standard treatments such as talk therapy or medications.

How can mind-body practices such as breathwork reach places in the mind where words cannot go? Here we share with you the story of Cholene Espinoza, a courageous woman who had always been a person of strong convictions, a practicing Christian, a true patriot, a caring person, and a loving friend. As a U.S. Air Force pilot, Cholene had been the second woman ever approved to fly a U-2 spy plane. After she left the air force, she worked as a commercial pilot for United Airlines. She was scheduled to be on Flight 93 on September 11, 2001, while commuting to another flight. When that flight was cancelled at the last minute, she had no reason to board Flight 93. However, her close friend from the U.S. Air Force Academy, the pilot Leroy Homer Jr., died when Flight 93 was hijacked by terrorists and crashed, leaving her with extreme survivor guilt.

Every incident is the result of a chain of events. Because she'd had intensive combat training in the air force, Cholene believed that if she had been on Flight 93, she might have sensed the presence of the terrorists and perhaps broken the fatal chain of events. After the September 11 disaster she felt helpless, angry, and disconnected from everyone and everything she had believed in. Hoping to regain her sense of connection to life, she did three tours as an embedded journalist in Iraq, starting with the U.S. Marine Corps 1st Tank Battalion during the invasion. She wants to tell her story of disconnection after the events of September 11 in her own words because she believes that her example may be of benefit to others affected by a mass disaster:

> Each time I returned from Iraq I felt that my world was meaning-less. There was a glass wall between my life and me, as I had known it. The institutions that I had been connected to, identified with and perhaps even defined myself by were like a hoax that never really existed—reality had shattered my image of life and my role in it. I was happiest when I was flying away and above it all, or running, or back in Iraq.
>
> I also threw myself into community service to regain a sense of purpose, devoting two years to post-Katrina work and helping to build a resource center in Mississippi, but this left me drained and still unable to feel joy or a sense of accomplishment.
>
> As time went on my desire to disconnect from the world grew. But, when faced with so much need in the world as I traveled to war zones in the Middle East as well as throughout Africa and India, I felt compelled to come out of my "bunker." The sense of duty to others was stronger than the desire to escape. Ironically, the pursuit of medicine satisfied both my need to be isolated and my desire to be of service. While studying for medical school I would have an excuse to isolate myself in order to become a physician. So, at the age of forty, I started a program of pre-med courses.

Leaving aviation, however, was like the death of my father. In the first few weeks of classes I kept reliving my days as a cadet at the Air Force Academy when my father died. I had difficulty focusing on my studies. I had not taken science courses in over twenty-two years. It felt like I was drowning. A close friend suggested that I could improve my mental focus by attending a breathing workshop.[6]

In September 2009, eight years after the terrorist attacks of September 2001, Cholene participated in one of our Breath~Body~Mind workshops, hoping it would help her relax and concentrate. During the afternoon breath practices on the first day of our workshop, she had a transformative experience of reconnection, which she shared with us:

The breathing and the rhythm of the bells were like the tide in the Arabian Gulf. The sound of the tide and the feel of the waves rolling over me were the only things that made me feel connected to life. The breathing was that and much more powerful because I was physically and mentally connecting to a larger energy source.

I found myself weeping when Dr. Brown said, "Think of those you love." I came away with a sense of being reunited with my life and loved ones. For the first time in years, I wanted to be connected to something besides a war or a disaster zone. After the breathing, during the meditation, I felt connected to the universe and to everyone in it.

Eight years after the terrorist attacks, Choline had recovered her sense of meaningful connection through breathwork. She continued to practice the breathing techniques as the benefits continued. She wrote to us later about her progress:

I am getting that focus. I just took midterms and, while I have a long way to go, I can see an enormous difference in these last two weeks versus the first two weeks of school. I feel a lightness and joy. I have always outwardly maintained a happy face to the world, but inwardly I struggled. Now the external and internal are in sync, like with the breathing. I feel a sense of connection with my family and friends that I have not felt in several years. While I still want to pursue medicine, it is not to isolate myself; nor is it completely out of a sense of duty. My desire to pursue medicine is out of a pure love of the knowledge and the possibility of having the privilege to share and apply that knowledge.

When she wrote this, Cholene was in her second year of medical school. She had found the way back to her true self and to her sense of connection with others. Joy in relationships, joy in work, and joy in being who we are . . . that's what life should be about.

Restoring a Sense of Bonding

In some cases, intensive psychotherapy can restore the sense of trust and bonding, but to our knowledge there are no medicines yet available that can restore the sense of bonding. Perhaps someday it will be possible to use prosocial hormone preparations such as oxytocin or other new discoveries to augment psychotherapy and other treatments. Most pharmaceutical research has focused on medications to dampen the sympathetic system to reduce anxiety and overreactivity rather than to boost the parasympathetic system or to stimulate oxytocin release. Hopefully, that will change now that the importance of the parasympathetic nervous system is being recognized.

Post-Traumatic Stress Disorder and Sexual Trauma

Sexual trauma can lead to post-traumatic stress disorder and can cause lifelong symptoms, particularly if untreated. Many victims of sexual abuse, especially children, are afraid to disclose what has happened or to ask for help. They may be left feeling unsafe, damaged, defective, and isolated even when they are with people who love and care for them. Research has shown that people with post-traumatic stress disorder can have dysfunction in their stress-response systems and in the brain circuits and anatomical structures responsible for processing fear, anger, and other emotions, particularly if the trauma occurred during childhood. This can include misperceptions of situations, distorted body image, fear of closeness, disconnection, anxiety, depression, and abnormal reactions such as overreactivity. The parts of the brain (particularly the prefrontal cortex and the insular cortex) that normally control the overactivity of the brain's emotion processing centers (the amygdala and hippocampus) become underactive. Consequently, the brain has less control of fear reactions, which results in the release of defensive reactions, as though the person feels that their life is in danger. These reactions can include trembling, rapid heartbeat, rapid breathing, a "knot" in the stomach, nausea, sweating, panic attacks, or numbing.

When frightened, some animals, for example rabbits, hold very still while watching carefully for a chance to escape. This is called a "freeze" reaction. Other animals, such as the possum, go limp and "play dead." Trauma victims can also react to perceived threats by freezing, feeling unable to move. When fighting or running away are both impossible, as is all too often the case with victims of abuse, their nervous system goes into a default mode, reverting to older circuits. This causes the person to feel paralyzed. The body becomes immobile and the speech centers shut down. When something or someone reminds the trauma survivor of the past abuse, the person may be triggered to respond by freezing and being unable to speak.

A woman we'll call Lisa sought treatment with Dr. Gerbarg. She had been sexually abused between the ages of three and ten, but never told anyone until she began psychotherapy at the age of twenty-nine. She finally sought help because despite being very physically attractive and personally appealing, she was lonely, depressed, and unable to find a husband. The story that emerged during treatment was that an older cousin had repeatedly molested her during family visits. As a result, she was terrified of men. Whenever she tried to talk to men, she froze. She learned to cover up this social paralysis by pretending to be aloof. Furthermore, because the abuse had been so painful, the thought of sexual intercourse petrified her, and she also felt that the molestation had permanently damaged her genitals, even though there was nothing visibly wrong. Feeling terrified, paralyzed, and defective, she was understandably unable to date or form a relationship with a man. Yet she longed for marriage and children.

In the course of a long psychotherapy, Lisa overcame her sense of shame enough to tell her family and her closest friends about the abuse. She developed deeper, more trusting relationships with women. Her self-esteem improved and with it her ability to take better care of herself. Overall, she was much happier, but she was still unable to date men. She was comfortable with male friends as long as they were no threat either because they were solidly married or homosexual.

At that time we were starting to study breath practices. Thinking that learning to do breathwork might help Lisa relax enough to begin dating, Dr. Gerbarg suggested she take the workshop. Being a highly motivated person, Lisa completed the workshop and for the next six months she practiced the breathing exercises every day for thirty minutes. She found that the practices took her to a place where she felt calm and peaceful. Dr. Gerbarg advised her to take the breathing workshop again, and she did. Afterward, in a therapy session, she talked about her healing experience: "During the breathing I felt a warm tingling sensation in the genital area. It felt like something was healing and I was no longer afraid."

During the next months, Lisa met and dated several men. She developed a deep relationship with one of them, George. He was very caring and supportive when she discussed her past traumas. As her trust in George grew, she felt ready for sexual intimacy. She harbored some worries about how she might react. She did not want to panic or freeze or have a flashback of the abuse. But whatever might happen, she knew she could depend on George to help her. When the time was right they made love.

To Lisa's surprise, her responses were completely normal and she thoroughly enjoyed it. In fact, they both thoroughly enjoyed making love every day, and at last report they were living together happily ever after.

How Breathing May Resolve Trauma

Seeing how the sexual trauma of Dr. Gerberg's patient Lisa had resolved with breathwork, we realized that we were witnessing something unexpected and extraordinary. Her transformation challenged us to figure out how breath practices could have dissolved the trauma formations, and corrected the distorted body perceptions and dysfunctional fear-processing circuits that had controlled Lisa's life for twenty-five years. We began by developing a neurophysiological model that could explain what we were seeing. The first part of the model consisted of the vagal nerve connections between the body and the brain's emotion regulatory centers and the effects of breath practices on the stress-response systems and fear circuits.[7] This could account for the damping down of Lisa's overreactivity and fear. The role of oxytocin in bonding added another dimension to the model. However, we needed to extend the model to explain how the practice of breath techniques could restore to normal the sensation and subjective experience of the genitals.

The missing pieces were found in work by Bud Craig, a neuroanatomist who is the director of the Atkinson Pain Research Laboratory and research professor in psychology at Arizona State University. Dr. Craig's research on the representation of feelings from the body has led to his theories on interoception: that is, the perception of the internal state of the body.[8] While the feelings on the outside of the body are processed in the somatosensory cortex, feelings from the inside of the body are processed in the interoceptive cortex, according to Craig. Interoceptions include feelings from the internal organs and tissues—for example, nausea, stomach pain, fullness, menstrual cramps, air hunger, vibrations, and many more. These internal sensations travel from the body up to the brain through the vagus nerves and eventually reach the interoceptive cortex, which lies deep within the sylvian fissure between the frontal and temporal lobes.

Once the information is received by the insular cortex, it undergoes higher level processing. For example, the interoceptive information has to be "perceived." Two people looking at the same painting will form two different subjective impressions of that painting. In a similar way, each person has a subjective way of experiencing interoceptive information from the body, and this is influenced by past experiences, current mental and emotional conditions, and the current hormonal and neurochemical milieu. This occurs all the time. Think about how your subjective perceptions and evaluations change depending on whether you are in a good or a bad mood, whether you have eaten recently or not, whether you feel tired or rested, and for women, where you are in your menstrual cycle. The subjective perception of interoceptive messages could help explain the drastic change in Lisa's perception of her genitals.

Because sexual trauma involves intense physical discomfort, the sensations from the body parts that were affected can become embedded in the trauma memories and formations. The subjective experience of sensations coming from that body part becomes distorted. In Lisa's case this was manifest in her feeling of genital damage. When Lisa did breath practices, there was no physical change in her genitals, yet there was a marked change in her subjective experience of those body parts. If we believe Craig's model, then it is possible that the interoceptive messages generated by the breath practices combined with changes in neurotransmitter activity and hormone levels induced changes in the interoceptive cortical connections. This could result in a shift in the subjective perception of her genitals and a reset to normal perceptions.

While the addition of Craig's work on interoception to our neurophysiological model provides a framework for understanding the power of breathing to resolve trauma, it is not enough. A model must be tested and reevaluated in light of new discoveries. More recently, we have been exploring the action of the brain's primary inhibitory neurotransmitter, gamma-aminobutyric acid (GABA), within the circuits that process trauma, fear, and the physical and emotional symptoms of post-traumatic stress disorder. Dr. Chris Streeter, an associate professor of psychiatry at Boston University Medical School has shown that a yoga practice can increase brain levels of GABA as measured with magnetic resonance spectroscopy, or MRS.[9] With Dr. Streeter, we hope to explore the effects of breathing and other mind-body practices on levels of GABA within the brain structures and circuits that process and regulate trauma-related emotions and their expression as symptoms in post-traumatic stress disorder.

Back to the Heart

We have come full circle. Starting with the capacity of the true self for love, bonding, and relationships we explored the effects of negative experiences and trauma on the brain and on stress-response systems in particular. By causing imbalances in stress-response systems and dysfunctions in emotion processing and regulation, trauma can disconnect us from our true selves, from others, and from the world around us. Breathing practices have the power to restore a healthy balance in the stress-response system, to unlock the grip of trauma on the mind and emotions, to create the conditions necessary for healing from the many effects of trauma. As this healing occurs, we rediscover our true selves and the capacity for love and bonding that are essential to our relationships.

7

Peak Performance

Use Your Breath to Change Your Life

> And as we let our own light shine, we unconsciously give other people permission to do the same.
>
> —*Marianne Williamson*, A Return to Love

We have shown you many of the ways that breath practices can be used to reduce the adverse effects of stress on your emotions and on your physical health. Breathwork can help relieve symptoms of everyday worry, anxiety, insomnia, depression, post-traumatic stress disorder, or physical injury. It can be used alone or as a complementary treatment that fits seamlessly into any therapeutic plan without causing side effects. And beyond improving stress resilience, breath practices can restore your sense of being genuinely who you are, of knowing what you feel, of recognizing what others feel, and of being able to experience deep and meaningful connections with people, with your values, and with all that is.

Breathing can be used for more than just healing injuries or solving problems. You can also enlist these techniques to help you achieve peak performance in all aspects of your life, including work, school, creative and artistic activities, and athletic performance.

Peak Performance through Breathing

What does it take to be the best one can be or to do the best one can do? Whether your goals are academic, athletic, artistic, or interpersonal, focusing your efforts and harmonizing your mind, body, and spirit will elevate your performance. Notice that we are not talking about being better than everyone else or being the best in the world. We are focusing on being the best that you can be with both your strengths and your weaknesses. Everyone has talents, but just wanting and trying are not enough. If you have honestly and consistently tried to reach a particular goal but still feel that you are not doing the best that you can do, it is possible that something is holding you back.

Breath practices can relieve the anxiety and tension that interfere with performance in any arena. They promote better integration of the mind, body, and emotions, enabling artistic expression to flow and optimizing physical movements to conserve energy and reduce wear and tear on joints, muscles, and tendons. And finally, the regular practice of Coherent Breathing or Resonant Breathing has been shown to improve circulation, oxygenation, and endurance.

Performance Anxiety

One of the most common blocks to achievement is anxiety and the tension it causes. This is as obvious in sports as it is in the performing arts. The basketball player who tenses up at the last minute is unlikely to sink his shot. The musician whose arms and shoulders tighten up will deliver a stilted performance. Every student knows that test anxiety can make the mind go blank. Learning to dissolve anxiety by breathing slowly, smoothly, and evenly can go a long way toward improving performance in any field of endeavor.

Disconnection or lack of integration can also impede performance.

Smooth, efficient actions require awareness and coordination of the mind, emotions, and body that includes both the performer and the instrument or the athlete and the sports equipment. The skier must be one with the skis just as the pianist must be one with the piano.

Wisdom from a Concert Pianist

Zita Zohar is an internationally renowned concert pianist. Through her years of coaching professional musicians and aspiring performers, she has developed a deep, intuitive understanding of the physical and emotional blocks that can interfere with performance. She has applied her knowledge of musical performance, neuroanatomy, and mind-body concepts to rehabilitate injured musicians as well as to enable performing artists to overcome blocks and to perform at their best.

Ms. Zohar is a master teacher who believes that breathing is intrinsic to musical performance. "All music tries to emulate the human voice and a voice needs time to breathe," she notes. "Both language and music are organized internally through breathing. Since both speech and music have phrases and pauses, breathing is essential to musical communication. If the performer is too nervous and stops breathing properly, the underlying message becomes unintelligible."

Ms. Zohar finds that nervousness is inherent during public performances. When musicians learn how to use slow, paced breathing while practicing and before starting a performance, the breathing serves to organize the brain and the body to move in tandem with the musical message. She encourages students to use Coherent Breathing for five to ten minutes before practicing their instrument. Many are overloaded with work and at first they feel they don't have much time for the breathwork, but it is difficult for them to refuse to do just five minutes. The students soon discover that those five minutes improve their concentration and the quality of their playing, but they need more, so they gradually increase their breath practice time. After about six months, many of them do the breathing for twenty minutes before each practice session and prior to performances.

A twenty-three-year-old music teacher named Emily had been studying with Ms. Zohar for two years. Although Emily had been playing piano since the age of six, she still felt anxious before performances. Sometimes her hands shook, engendering a fear that she might lose control of her performance. At Ms. Zohar's suggestion, she attended a Breath~Body~Mind workshop in February 2011. Emily later summed up her thoughts about incorporating breath practice into her musical life:

> One of the greatest changes I feel after breathing and meditating is a sense of renewed energy and clarity of the mind; as if I've woken up from a deep and restful sleep. Sometimes it is possible to lose track of time when meditating, as my mind goes into another state. After a good breathing and meditation session, I'm able to practice for longer sessions more effectively without getting tired of repetition, an inherent aspect of practicing. After a particularly restful meditation, I feel more centered and calm. When I feel calmer, the music flows better and I feel like I'm so much more emotionally connected to the piano, more focused and able to keep the goal I am trying to achieve clearly in my mind. The music becomes more expressive. The next challenge is that with continued meditation practice, I will be able to achieve this "knowing calm" not just during practice, but also during performances.

According to Ms. Zohar, antiquated systems of teaching neglect the incorporation of correct body positioning and breath training. Body tension and incorrect positioning can result in injuries such as carpal tunnel syndrome and dystonia, a painful condition of chronic excess muscle tension and spasm. The methods to prevent and correct such problems, especially when teaching children, need to be improved to include the support of the entire body both in practicing and in public performance.

The rate of injury of musicians of all ages is being recognized as a significant problem, and there is increasing acceptance that changes are necessary. The realization that each movement should produce the desired effect efficiently and with the least physical strain brings to the fore the importance of the relationship between the musician's stress, her body, and her instrument. When people are under stress, their breathing becomes shallow and their shoulders tend to go upward. This creates tension and changes the alignment of the body with the instrument such that the body is not properly supported, leading to fatigue, strain, and impaired performance. A musician's use of Coherent Breathing can alleviate tension and enable the shoulders to stay down. At the same time, the body thus becomes more grounded. The optimal use of all available support, not only the support of the torso by the chair but also the hands touching the instrument and the feet resting on the floor, enhances the focus and control of the performance.

Resistance Breathing with Coherent Breathing helps relieve the high anxiety that plagues many performers. Students gain confidence once they realize that they have the ability to control anxiety by using breathing techniques. Ms. Zohar incorporates breath practices with Feldenkrais techniques, which focus on the relationship between physical movement and thought, mental awareness, and creativity (www.feldenkrais.com). The integration of breathing and body movements, along with their effects on the musician's interaction with the instrument, is particularly helpful for performers and students who have become disconnected through years of misguided use of their body. Ms. Zohar observes, "When used properly, the human body has incredible capabilities to participate in creative efforts. It is possible, using breathing techniques and Feldenkrais, to restore the natural synergistic connections between the performing artist's body, the musical instrument, and the creative process to produce an artistically worthwhile statement."

Music performance anxiety, which occurs in about 25 percent of musicians, has a strongly adverse effect on the entire spectrum of musicianship, including the general physical and emotional well-being of musicians as well as on their career choices and quality of performance.[1] Although nonprofessional music students face less pressure, they can still be vulnerable to similar anxiety-producing forces. Tens of thousands of students take music lessons or participate in school bands and orchestras. Most are expected to perform solo as well as in groups. By increasing understanding and awareness of the effects of stress and anxiety, parents, teachers, and students can develop more effective coping strategies using movement, breathing, and meditation techniques. This would help to reduce strain and injury as well as anxiety. Without fear or anxiety, the musician can be freed to enjoy the art of making music—and the same potential for freedom from anxiety applies to all creative and performance arts, such as dancing, acting, painting, and writing. Coherent Breathing, Resistance Breathing, and Breath Moving can remove obstacles to peak artistic performance.

Anxiety and Athletics: Two Sides of the Coin

Athletes striving for a peak performance are certainly familiar with the fine line between excitement and anxiety. Some level of manageable anxiety stimulates adrenaline and heightens alertness for competition. However, when anxiety becomes too intense, it can undermine athletic performance by creating excess muscular tension, impairing fine motor control, and causing shallow breathing. For peak athletic performance, we recommend twenty to sixty minutes per day of breathing at five to six breaths per minute and ten to twenty minutes of similar breath practice just prior to sports activities. This will prepare the muscles with an ample supply of blood and oxygen from the very start of the action. It will also help to control interference from excess anxiety or tension. This is an effective way to remove obstacles to peak performance.

The average person can hold their breath for three to four minutes. *Hypoxia* refers to an insufficiency in the level of oxygen in the bloodstream. *Hypercapnia* refers to an excessive level of carbon dioxide in the bloodstream. When the oxygen level drops too low or when the carbon dioxide level rises too high, sensors called chemoreceptors tell the brain that the body needs to take another breath, but training with slow-paced breathing can reduce the sensitivity of chemoreceptors to hypoxia and hypercapnia.

The result is that the person is able to comfortably tolerate lower levels of oxygen without feeling the need to take another breath as quickly. Intense exercise consumes oxygen rapidly, exposing body tissues to low levels of oxygen. This can lead to tissue damage unless the oxygen supply increases or the need for oxygen decreases by reducing the intensity of exercise.

There are many situations in which it is advantageous to be able to tolerate hypoxia and hypercapnia. Here are just a few.

1. Deep-water divers can learn to hold their breath for up to seven minutes.
2. Musicians who play wind instruments can hold their notes longer.
3. Singers can keep singing for longer periods of time before having to pause for breath.
4. Athletes can increase endurance and keep playing longer before feeling short of breath.
5. The body can recover faster after exercise.
6. People skiing or hiking in the mountains are less likely to develop high-altitude sickness.

High-Altitude Performance

To study the cardiovascular effects of high altitudes, an Italian professor of cardiology studied a group of professional mountain climbers who practiced breathing at six breaths per minute one hour daily for two years before attempting to climb Mount Everest, whose peak is at 29,035 feet (8,850 meters) above sea level. The cardiologist, Dr. Luciano Bernardi, compared the performance of those climbers with that of a group of professional climbers who had not practiced the breathing. Dr. Bernardi found that climbers who did the breath training reached the summit without auxiliary oxygen and with a respiratory rate of only ten breaths per minute. In contrast, the other climbers needed to use oxygen tanks and struggled to breathe at the peak.[2] In general, people use only about 20 percent of the surface area of their lungs, that is, the inner surface that lines the alveoli, the millions of air sacs that exchange oxygen and carbon dioxide with the bloodstream. The climbers who had practiced breathing at six breaths per minute for a year were able to use 80 percent of the surface of their lungs, the maximum possible area for oxygen exchange. Since they were able to extract much more oxygen from the air with each breath, they could take in an adequate amount of oxygen by breathing more slowly.

Dr. Bernardi made an additional discovery about the effects of paced breathing on peripheral circulation. Muscle strength and endurance depend on robust circulation to supply oxygen and remove lactic acid. Lactic acid causes muscle pain, cramps, and, if prolonged, damage to muscle tissues. Slow-paced breathing can increase circulation, oxygenation, and removal of toxic byproducts such as lactic acid. Dr. Bernardi found that a respiratory rate of six breaths per minute caused the capillaries (tiny blood vessels) in the hands and feet to dilate, resulting in maximal blood flow to the extremities.

You don't have to be a professional mountain climber to benefit from paced-breath training, as one of our friends discovered. Janice and her husband loved adventurous vacations. A few weeks before traveling to Colorado, Janice took our Breath~Body~Mind workshop, but between then and her trip she felt too busy to practice Coherent Breathing. At the last minute before leaving for vacation, however, she tossed a *Respire-1* CD into her backpack. On her second day in Colorado, while staying at a resort about ten thousand feet above sea level, she became ill with a throbbing headache, dizziness, nausea, weakness, and lethargy — classic symptoms of high-altitude sickness. Somehow, through her brain fog, she remembered the CD, dug it out of her backpack, popped it into her CD player, and slowed herself down to five breaths per minute. Within half an hour she was feeling better. For the remainder of their vacation, Janice used Coherent Breathing every day to prevent a recurrence of the high-altitude sickness.

Golf: A Game of Nerves

Golf is one of those games that require intense mental concentration and simultaneous physical relaxation to perform smooth, powerful, accurate strokes. Too much anxiety and the golfer will tense up, throwing off his or her swing. Tom had the talent to become a pro golfer, but whenever he entered competition, his anxiety would rise and ruin his game. Finally, he sought psychiatric help. During Tom's second visit to Dr. Gerbarg's office, she taught him some slow Resistance Breathing exercises to use whenever he was waiting to step up to the tee. Tom found that the breathing practice kept his anxiety in check, allowing him to play at a level consistent with his real abilities. He succeeded in qualifying to be a pro golf instructor and to enter the tournaments that were crucial for his career. He said a thankful good-bye at his third and final visit, then headed south for his new job as the golf pro at a beautiful country club.

Warrior-Healers and Athletes

People who participate in contact and combat sports inevitably experience major and minor injuries. In traditional martial arts, warriors are trained in techniques to reduce the risk of injury as well as ways to quickly repair whatever damage occurs. Intense breath training is an essential part of this preparation because it increases strength and endurance and sharpens the awareness that is necessary to counterattacks and evade blows.

BREATH PRACTICES IN AIKIDO

Aikido is a Japanese martial art whose primary purpose is spiritual development and the restoration of harmony in the universe through the use of qi, the life force. The concept of aikido is that when someone attacks they disturb the harmony of the universe. By countering or neutralizing the attack, aikido restores the harmony. Training includes many hours of physical exercises, meditation, and breathing sessions using different rates and intensities. Advanced practitioners learn to breathe as slowly as one breath per minute. Dr. Brown has studied aikido for twenty-five years with Sensei Imaizumi and became an aikido teacher at the fourth-dan level. At that level breathing is used to develop enough endurance and situational awareness to fend off five attackers at once. Trainees also learn to use a very deep, loud, sharp shout to prime their bodies for sudden strong movements. This training came in handy one summer when Dr. Brown was called upon to help clear some land by throwing fallen trees into a ravine. Each time he lifted a heavy trunk, he let loose with a mighty shout that soared out over the lake below as he flung trees over the cliff into the chasm. The other men on his crew were impressed, and they quickly learned how to use his technique. The men were up there all day, shouting and heaving. That evening after they returned for dinner, the phone rang. Apparently their shouts had carried for miles and miles, all the way across the lake, terrifying the residents and tourists. Fortunately, their job was done and from that night on no shouts disturbed the peace of the lake.

QIGONG MASTER ROBERT PENG

Qigong training has many physical and spiritual dimensions. When the qigong master Robert Peng (whom we already mentioned in chapter 5) was training with his Shaolin master, he was given the choice of developing his skills for combat or for healing. Although he chose healing, he also trained in many techniques used to fortify the body. Among the skills he acquired, Master Peng developed the ability to focus enough energy through his fingers to generate electrical currents, which he uses for healing. Another skill he teaches is to increase "guardian qi," energy that increases the body's resistance to illness or injury. For example, using this energy, the body resists being pierced by sharp objects and when it receives a hard blow, no bruise will develop. Master Peng teaches many different breath practices including a kind of Resistance Breathing in which the breath is moved through partially clenched teeth and Longevity Walking, which synchronizes Breath Counts with walking. Those who are interested in such techniques can read Master Peng's account of his life, *Qigong Master: My Life and Secret Teachings,*[3] and visit his Web site, www.robert peng.com, for his schedule of workshops and a list of his training DVDs.

A Brief Reprise

We have seen that breath practices, especially Coherent and Resonant Breathing, remove obstacles such as anxiety and muscle tension, enabling creativity to be expressed and flow more easily from artists through their instruments. You will find that the regular use of breathing practices can improve your level of mental, physical, and artistic performance. By reducing tension, alleviating anxiety, and improving blood flow and oxygenation, breathing practices enhance speed, accuracy, strength, and endurance.

8

Conclusion and Review of Breathing Practices

E ven though you have read this far, you still may not fully realize that you now have the ability to change your life by using the breathing and movement practices you have learned. We are going to review the practices and the many ways they can be useful. At first, you may want a summary guide to keep track of the indications, timing, and benefits of each practice. For a quick reference to the breath practices, see table 1 in the appendix, "How and When to Use Each Practice." After the review of breathing and movement practices that follows, we will show you how to go even further to attain peak performance at work, at home, and in creative, artistic, and athletic performance.

The Total Breath: Coherent Breathing, Resistance Breathing, and Breath Moving

Coherent Breathing sets the fundamental rhythm for transformation. If you use only one technique from this book, let it be Coherent Breathing.

The tracks on the *Healing Power of the Breath* CD that accompanies this book are used to pace your breathing to either five or six breaths per minute. This simple, gentle, versatile practice should be done at least once a day with full concentration—that is, with eyes closed and either sitting or reclining. For best effects, for most people, at least twenty minutes of uninterrupted Coherent Breathing works well. However, there is no limit on the length of this practice: the more you do it, the better you will feel. If you are dealing with intense stress, anxiety, depression, PTSD, pain, or medical illness, then you may need to do the practice twenty minutes twice a day.

After about three months of concentrated practice, additional time doing Coherent Breathing with eyes open can be added on and off throughout the day. Do as much as you like to prevent a buildup of stress and to relieve anxiety. As the table in the appendix indicates, Coherent Breathing can relieve stress, tension, anxiety, worry, phobias, insomnia, and respiratory problems. By increasing parasympathetic activity and decreasing sympathetic activity, Coherent Breathing balances and stabilizes the stress-response system, helping you to react more appropriately rather than with excess fear, anger, or feelings of helpless immobility. The increased parasympathetic activity calms the mind, slows the heart, lowers blood pressure, reduces inflammation, and strengthens stress resilience.

Resistance Breathing is used to augment Coherent Breathing. Whether you choose to make a sound in the back of your throat like the ocean or to use pursed lips to create resistance to the flow of air, your practice of Resistance Breathing can amplify the benefits of Coherent Breathing.

Breath Moving entails moving the breath in circuits to different parts of the body, moving upward on the inhale and downward on the exhale. Adding Breath Moving to Coherent Breathing and Resistance Breathing enhances the benefits of those breath practices. Breath Moving circulates energy and can be used to elevate energy as well as to relieve pain.

When you combine Coherent Breathing, Resistance Breathing, and Breath Moving into one single practice, we call it the Total Breath.

The Complete Practice: Movement, Breathing, and Meditation or Relaxation

For the best breathwork practice, we suggest that you do a complete sequence of movement, breathing, and meditation (or relaxation) when time allows. Yoga, qigong, tai chi, and warm-up or stretching exercises remove a layer of physical tension before starting the breathing techniques. In addition, such movements improve joint health, flexibility, and joint mobility, and they help relieve muscle tension and pain in the joints or muscles.

For relaxation, try the body scans we have given you in chapter 1. If you have only a few minutes, you can place your attention on your feet, ankles, knees, elbows, abdomen, chest, neck, head, and whole body. If you have more time, you can linger longer and feel your pulse in more places. Taking more time deepens the relaxation experience. Resting for even a few minutes, lying on your right side at the end of the Complete Practice, allows your nervous system to consolidate and remember what you have experienced. This is important for building up the benefits of practice over time.

"Ha" Breath, Breath Counting, 4-4-6-2 Breathing, and Breath Moving

Rather than write an exhaustive book with hundreds of breath practices, we have selected a few that are easy to teach, easy to learn, safe, rapidly effective, and useful in many different aspects of life. These can be done separately or after the movements and before Coherent Breathing as part of the Complete Practice.

"Ha" Breath is good for relieving mental fatigue, inattention, attention deficit disorder, and fuzzy thinking. It tends to energize while it increases mental focus, concentration, and attention. One to five minutes of "Ha" Breath should be sufficient for these purposes.

Counting each phase of the breath using 4-4-6-2 is as effective today as it was in ancient times for quieting the mind and for reducing anger and impulsivity. Combining 4-4-6-2 breath counting with movements is even more effective for banishing intrusive negative thoughts such as thoughts of suicide.

Vibration Breathing

Chanting *om* is calming, soothing, and balancing. The vibrations stimulate the vagus nerve and the parasympathetic system as well as internal organs and body tissues. *Om* engenders peaceful feelings by harmonizing the mind, body, and spirit.

Master Robert Peng teaches that the sound of chanting *song, kong, tong, dong* increases insight, clarity, and mental focus. Thus, it is especially helpful when you are feeling scattered, unsettled, unfocused, agitated, or overwhelmed.

Breathing while moving and stretching is good for muscle tension or pain in the neck, back, muscles, or joints. Coherent Breathing enhanced with Resistance Breathing can be done with most movement sequences to increase flexibility, joint mobility, and endurance. It may also reduce inflammation, prevent damage, and support the healing of injuries.

How Will Breathing Practices Change Your Life?

Breath practices have changed the lives of millions of people. How they will change your life depends on the effort you put into learning and practicing some of the methods in this book as well as attending more intensive courses. While this book and the *Healing Power of the Breath* CD were created for your individual use at home, we recognize that learning and doing all of this on your own can be challenging. Maintaining the motivation and commitment to doing the practices regularly, ideally every day, is also difficult. Most people find that taking our two-day Breath~Body~Mind workshop brings about intense, deep changes more rapidly. Also, the support of others in the workshop and follow-up sessions can bolster your motivation.

The basic Breath~Body~Mind workshop usually runs for twelve hours over two consecutive days. This immersion allows people to experience a sequence of rounds, with each round consisting of movement, breathing, and meditation or relaxation. With each round, layers of stress are removed and the corrective effects of the practices become deeper and more powerful. While most people feel much better after the workshop, those who do the practices regularly over time accrue the greatest benefits. Remember, it takes time to rebalance the stress-response system and it takes time to rewire old patterns of emotional response. You need to put aside the endless distractions and tasks of your busy life so that you can focus attention on what goes on inside of you.

It also takes time to develop a more subtle awareness of the sensations in one's body, the thoughts in one's mind, and the feelings in one's heart. Your life will change as you free yourself from reactions to past hurts, cultivate positive emotions, and restore your sense of peace and safety. The more you become aware and accepting of your inner world, the better you will be able to see clearly what you need to do, remove obstacles to your growth, and care lovingly for yourself and others. Ultimately, it is well worth the time and effort to become reunited with your true self.

Acknowledgments

The Healing Power of the Breath has many roots, some from ancient mind-body-spirit practices, some from modern neuroscience, psychology, and physiology, and others from our more than thirty years of clinical practice in psychiatry. We have many mentors to thank for preparing us with the knowledge to investigate the use of breathing practices in the treatment of medical and psychological problems. In addition, we are thankful for the many friends and colleagues who contributed to the writing and editing of this book.

Dr. Brown honors the teachers who transmitted to him their knowledge of ancient practices as well as their own innovations. Sensei Shizuo Imaizumi is one of the few living masters trained by the founder of aikido, Morihei Ueshiba. In 1986 Sensei Imaizumi first introduced Dr. Brown to coherent breathing. He also honors the Seido karate master and Zen teacher Tadashi Nakumura; Satguru, Sri Sri Ravi Shankar, the creator of Sudarshan Kriya Yoga; Les Fehmi, PhD, a Zen teacher and one of the fathers of biofeedback who discovered Open Focus meditation; the qigong master T.K. Shi; and Master Robert Peng, who was chosen as a child for training in qigong by the Chinese Buddhist healing monk Xiao Yao, abbot of the Shaolin Temple. We especially thank Master Peng for allowing us to include his *song, kong, tong, dong* technique in chapter 5.

Next, we extend our appreciation to Stephen Elliot, who generously provided the beautiful chime sound tracks for the *Healing Power of the Breath* CD. Steve draws upon his experience as a qigong practitioner and his background in engineering to blend beautiful tones with precision timing in his works. Thanks also go to composer-musician Peter Einhorn of Unicorn Productions, who recorded and mastered the CD for us.

This book was greatly enhanced by three talented readers who gave invaluable critiques: Gretchen Wallace, Leslie Andrade, and Michele Whittemore. Gretchen, an Integrative Breathwork therapist, is the founder and president of Global Grassroots, a nonprofit organization that operates the Academy for Conscious Change, based in Rwanda. The academy teaches mind-body practices, conscious leadership, and social entrepreneurship to vulnerable women recovering from war and disaster in Africa. Gretchen taught Breath~Body~Mind practices to Haitian survivors of the 2010 earthquake, and she has incorporated Breath~Body~Mind into the programs for women in Rwanda. Leslie Andrade, MEd, is an elementary school teacher. We met her at a writer's workshop at Brown University and she has been editing our books ever since. By offering to be the first to use this book to learn breath practices, Leslie was able to point out places where clarification was needed and to raise many provocative questions. Michele Whittemore, MEd, teaches English at Ramapo High School in Franklin Lakes, New Jersey. She read our manuscript with her heart and brought out the emotional and spiritual intention.

For the past three years, Ellen Ratner, MEd, of Talk Radio news service, and Dr. Luka Deng of the Pamela Lipkin, MD, clinic in South Sudan have been using Breath~Body~Mind to relieve trauma in survivors of war and slavery. They welcomed our program and have given us feedback about the benefits they are seeing among the Sudanese.

We are deeply grateful to the many students who participated in our Breath~Body~Mind workshops and who contributed their stories to illustrate the many ways that breath practices can help people overcome challenges in their lives. In particular, we thank Cholene Espinoza for her service to our country as a pilot in the United States Air Force and for sharing her story of recovery from the September 11, 2001, terrorist attacks on the World Trade Center and the hijacking of Flight 93. By the time this book is published, Cholene will be well on her way toward graduating from medical school.

We wish to thank our dear friend, Zita Zohar, a master teacher and concert pianist, who graciously contributed her thoughts about the use of breath practices in the performing arts (see chapter 7). Emily Chou, one of her piano students, shared her use of breathwork to meet the challenge of performance anxiety.

We are grateful to the editors of Shambhala Publications, Beth Frankl and Ben Gleason, for working closely with us throughout the publication process. Their collaborative spirit and professionalism were most helpful. We also thank Wendy Carrel, our book shepherd, for helping to publicize our work.

Appendix

Table 1. How and When to Use Each Practice

Practice	Condition or Situation	Time of Day	Dose	Frequency	Effects
Coherent Breathing	Stress, tension, anxiety, worry, phobias, insomnia, medical illness, respiratory problems (may need to start with 6 bpm or more), performance	A.M. or P.M. Anytime	20 min. 5 min. up to an hour or more	Twice a day On and off throughout the day and continuously during periods of stress	Calm the mind, relax the body, reduce fear, restore sleep, balance stress-response systems, promote healing, prevent illness, progression, reduce pain, enhance performance
Resistance Breathing (Ocean Breath, ujjayi)	Use with Coherent Breathing on out-breaths to increase calming effects	A.M. or P.M. Anytime	Start with 5 min. and work up to 20 min.	Twice a day On and off throughout the day for stress	Same as Coherent Breathing

Practice	Condition or Situation	Time of Day	Dose	Frequency	Effects
Pursed lips	Use with Coherent Breathing on out-breaths when nasal passages are too blocked to breathe through nose	A.M. or P.M. Anytime	Start with 5 min. and work up to 20 min.	Twice a day On and off through-out the day for stress	Same as Coherent Breathing
Breath Moving	To increase effects of Coherent Breathing. Asthma (always move breath when doing Coherent Breathing), Attention Deficit Disorder (ADD), Pain	A.M. or P.M. unless it is overactivating at night Before and during study or work	5–20 min. As long as needed	Twice a day On and off through-out the day as needed	Same as Coherent Breathing. Helps maintain attention during breath practice. Can increase energy and reduce pain.

Practice	Condition or Situation	Time of Day	Dose	Frequency	Effects
Total Breath (Coherent Breathing + Resistance Breathing + Breath Moving)	To maximize effectiveness of breath practices and rapidity of response	A.M. or P.M. Anytime	5–20 min. As long as needed	Twice a day On and off throughout the day as needed	Strengthens all the effects of Coherent Breathing, Resistance Breathing, and Breath Moving
Body scan	Relaxes and connects mind and body	A.M. or P.M.	5–8 min.	After breath practices	Calms, soothes, relaxes, creates peaceful and connected feelings
Rest lying on right side	Allows mind and body to absorb the effects of the practices, eases transition back to normal activities	A.M. or P.M.	At least 1 min. 5 min. or longer if you have time	After breath practices and body scan	Integrates and consolidates effects of breath practices for more lasting results

Practice	Condition or Situation	Time of Day	Dose	Frequency	Effects
"Ha" Breath	Mental fatigue, inattention, ADD, fuzzy thinking	Before Coherent Breathing Use alone anytime	1–5 min.	Before Coherent Breathing Use alone for mental work	Increase energy, mental focus, concentration, and attention. Avoid if you have seizures, high blood pressure, aneurysm, recent surgery, or are pregnant.
Breath Counts 4-4-6-2	Stress, tension, anxiety, worry, intrusive or suicidal thoughts	Anytime	8–10 repetitions, 5–10 min.	After "Ha" Breath and before Coherent Breathing. Anytime for stopping unwanted thoughts.	Calms, soothes, balances. Reduces angry, violent, or suicidal thoughts. Reduces impulsivity.
Breath Counts + movement	Stress, tension, anxiety, worry, intrusive/ suicidal thoughts, muscle tension, pain in tendons or muscles	Add movements to 4-4-6-2 any time	4–10 repetitions, 5–10 min.	Move with 4-4-6-2 anytime. For stopping impulsivity, anger, suicidal thoughts.	Calms, soothes, balances. Increases effectiveness of 4-4-6-2. Reduces angry, violent, or suicidal thoughts. Reduces impulsivity.

Practice	Condition or Situation	Time of Day	Dose	Frequency	Effects
Vibration Breathing: *Om*	Stress, tension, anxiety, worry	After Breath Counts and before Coherent Breathing	3 repetitions Prolong the *om* sound as you exhale	Augment soothing and internal healing effects	Calms, soothes, balances. Stimulates internal organs and body tissues. Harmonizes mind and body. Creates peaceful feelings.
Vibration Breathing: *Song, kong, tong, dong*	Feeling scattered, unsettled, unfocused, agitated, overwhelmed	After Breath Counts and before Coherent Breathing	6–12 repetitions 3–6 min.	1–3 times/week or more as needed	Increases insight, clarity, mental focus. Recharges energy. Promotes nurturing feelings.
Song, kong, tong, dong + Breath Moving	Fatigue, feeling scattered, unsettled, unfocused, agitated, overwhelmed	After Breath Counts and before Coherent Breathing	9 rounds 5–7 min.	1–3 times/week or more as needed	Increases effects of *song, kong, tong, dong.* Increases and circulates energy, refreshes, harmonizes mind and body.

Practice	Condition or Situation	Time of Day	Dose	Frequency	Effects
Stretching + Coherent Breathing, Resistance Breathing, or both	Muscle tension; neck, back, muscle, or joint pain; carpal tunnel syndrome; performance	Before breath practices or use alone anytime	3 or more complete breaths for each stretch or joint	1 time/day or more if needed	Increases effectiveness of stretches. Increases flexibility and endurance. Reduces inflammation, pain. Helps heal injuries.
Stretching + Coherent Breathing, Resistance Breathing, or both + Breath Moving	Muscle, tendon, joint pain or injury. Move the breath through the area of pain.	Before breath practices or use alone anytime	3 or more complete breaths for each stretch or joint	1 time/day or more if needed	Increases circulation and relaxation in area of injury. Reduces pain and inflammation.

Table 2. Order of Practice

	Movement	"Ha" Breath	4-4-6-2 Breath + Movement	Joint Rotation + Breath	Om	Song, Kong, Tong, Dong	Breathing	Meditation or Relaxation	Rest
A.M. 20 min.	Yoga or other warm-up stretches, Qigong movements or tai chi						Total Breath (Coherent Breathing + Resistance Breathing + Breath Moving)	Body scan, meditation, positive affirmations, or visualization	Lie on right side 5 min. or more
P.M. 20 min	Same as above if you have the time and energy						Coherent Breathing + Resistance Breathing	Body scan, meditation, positive affirmations, or visualization	Drift off to sleep

	Movement	"Ha" Breath	4-4-6-2 Breath + Movement	Joint Rotation + Breath	Om	Song, Kong, Tong, Dong	Breathing	Meditation or Relaxation	Rest
Mind wanders during breathing			Use 4-4-6-2				Use Breath Moving		
Tiredness during the day		2–5 min.							
Inattention		2–5 min.							
ADHD	Yoga, qigong, warm-up	2–5 min.	4-4-6-2 breathing + movement		3 times	9 times	Coherent Breathing + Resistance Breathing + Breath Moving	Body scan	Lie on right side 5 min. or more

	Movement	"Ha" Breath	4-4-6-2 Breath + Movement	Joint Rotation + Breath	Om	Song, Kong, Tong, Dong	Breathing	Meditation or Relaxation	Rest
Anxiety Worry Stress Insomnia	Yoga, qigong, or warm-up		5 min.		3 times	9 times	Total Breath, 20 min., twice daily + 5–20 min.	5–10 min.	5 min. or more
Depression PTSD Fibromyalgia	10 min., twice daily	2–5 min.	5 min.		3 times	9 times	Total Breath, 20 min., twice daily	Body scan 5–10 min.	5 min. or more
Anger			5–10 min.						
Suicidal thoughts			5–10 min.						
Sports	Flexibility		5 min.	Prevent injuries Heal injuries	3 times	9 times	Total Breath 10–20 min.	Body scan 5 min.	1–5 min.

	Movement	"Ha" Breath	4-4-6-2 Breath + Movement	Joint Rotation + Breath	Om	Song, Kong, Tong, Dong	Breathing	Meditation or Relaxation	Rest
Performance anxiety, stress, tension	Reduce body tension		5 min. before performance		3 times	9 times	Total Breath, 20 min. 1 or 2 times daily 10–20 min. before performing	5 min. during A.M. or P.M. practice	5 min. A.M. or P.M. practice

Notes

Chapter 1

1. Beauchaine, T. P., "Vagal Tone, Development, and Gray's Motivational Theory: Toward an Integrated Model of Autonomic Nervous System Functioning in Psychopathology," *Developmental Psychopathology* 13, no. 2 (2001): 183–214; Beauchaine, T. P., Katkin, E. S., Strassberg, Z., and Snarr, J., "Disinhibitory Psychopathology in Male Adolescents: Discriminating Conduct Disorder from Attention-Deficit/Hyperactivity Disorder through Concurrent Assessment of Multiple Autonomic States," *Journal of Abnormal Psychology* 110, no. 4 (2001): 610–624; Brown, R. P., and Gerbarg, P. L., "Sudarshan Kriya Yogic Breathing in the Treatment of Stress, Anxiety, and Depression: Part 1 — Neurophysiologic Model," *Journal of Alternative and Complementary Medicine* 11, no. 1 (2005): 189–201; Brown, R. P., Gerbarg, P. L., and Muskin, P. R., *How to Use Herbs, Nutrients, and Yoga in Mental Health Care* (New York: W. W. Norton, 2009); Porges, S. W., "The Polyvagal Theory: Phylogenetic Substrates of a Social Nervous System," *International Journal of Psychophysiology* 42, no. 2 (2001): 123–146.
2. Hassett, A. L., Radvanski, D. C., Vaschillo, E. G., Vaschillo, B., Sigal, L. H., Karavidas, M. K., Buyske, S., and Lehrer, P. M., "A Pilot Study of the Efficacy of Heart Rate Variability (HRV) Biofeedback in Patients with Fibromyalgia," *Applied Psychophysiology Biofeedback* 32, no. 1 (2007): 1–10.

3. Lehrer, P., Sasaki, Y., and Saito, Y., "Zazen and Cardiac Variability," *Psychosomatic Medicine* 61, no. 6 (1999): 812–821.
4. Bernardi, L., Sleight, P., Bandinelli, G., Cencetti, S., Fattorini, L., Wdowczyc-Szulc, J., and Lagi, A., "Effect of Rosary Prayer and Yoga Mantras on Autonomic Cardiovascular Rhythms: A Comparative Study," Health Module, *British Medical Journal* 323, no. 7327 (2001): 1446.
5. Elliot, S., and Edmonson, D., *Coherent Breathing: The Definitive Method, Theory, and Practice* (Allen, TX: Coherence Press, 2008).

Chapter 2

1. Brown, R. P., and Gerbarg, P. L., "Sudarshan Kriya Yogic Breathing, Part 1"; Brown, R. P., and Gerbarg, P. L., "Yoga Breathing, Meditation, and Longevity," in *Longevity, Regeneration, and Optimal Health* (Annals of the New York Academy of Sciences, vol. 1172), edited by C. Bushell, E. L. Olivo, and N. D. Theise (Boston, MA: Wiley-Blackwell, 2009); Calabrese, P., Perrault, H., Dinh, T. P., Eberhard, A., and Benchetrit, G., "Cardiorespiratory Interactions during Resistive Load Breathing," *American Journal of Physiology: Regulatory, Integrative, and Comparative Physiology* 279, no. 6 (2000): R2208–R2213.
2. Porges, S. W., "The Polyvagal Theory: New Insights into Adaptive Reactions of the Autonomic Nervous System," *Cleveland Clinic Journal of Medicine* 76, no. 2 (2009): S86–S90; Porges, "The Polyvagal Theory: Phylogenetic Substrates."
3. Yu, J., "Airway Mechanosensors," *Respiratory Physiology Neurobiology* 148, no. 3 (2005): 217–243.
4. Philippot, P., Gaetane, C., and Blairy, S., "Respiratory Feedback in the Generation of Emotion," *Cognition and Emotion* 16, no. 5 (2002): 605–607.

Chapter 3

1. Vasiliev, Vladimir, *Let Every Breath . . . Secrets of the Russian Breath Masters* (Richmond Hill, Ontario: Russian Martial Art, 2006).

Chapter 4

1. Brown, R. P., and Gerbarg, P. L., "Sudarshan Kriya Yogic Breathing, Part 1"; Brown, R. P., and Gerbarg, P. L., "Yoga Breathing, Meditation, and Longevity"; Kuntsevich, V., Bushell, W. C., and Theise, N. D., "Mechanisms of Yogic Practices in Health, Aging, and Disease," *Mount Sinai*

Journal of Medicine 77, no. 5 (2010): 559–569; Thayer, J. F., and Brosschot, J. F., "Psychosomatics and Psychopathology: Looking Up and Down from the Brain," *Psychoneuroendocrinology* 30, no. 10 (2005):1050–1058.

2. *Diagnostic and Statistical Manual* DSM-IV, 1994.
3. Katzman, M., et al., "A Multicomponent Yoga-Based, Breath Intervention Program as Adjunctive Treatment in Patients Suffering from Generalized Anxiety Disorder (GAD) with or without Comorbidities," paper presented at the Anxiety Disorders Association of America conference, Albuquerque, NM, March 10–12, 2009. This paper has just been submitted for publication.
4. Katzman, M., et al., "Breath-Body-Mind-Workshop as Adjunctive Treatment in Patients Suffering from Generalized Anxiety Disorder (GAD) with or without Comorbidity," paper presented at the American Psychiatric Association Annual Meeting, New Orleans, LA, May 22–23, 2010.
5. Brown, R. P., Gerbarg, P. L., Vermani, M., and Katzman, M., "First and Second Trials of Breathing, Movement, and Meditation PTSD, Depression, and Anxiety Related to September 11th New York City World Trade Center Attacks," lecture given at the annual meeting of the American Psychiatric Association, New Orleans, LA, May 22, 2010.
6. Brown et al., *How to Use Herbs, Nutrients, and Yoga in Mental Health Care.*
7. Gerbarg, P. L., Wallace, Gretchen S., and Brown, R. P., "Mass Disasters and Mind-Body Solutions for Mass Disasters: Evidence and Field Insights," *International Journal of Yoga Therapy* 21 (2011): 97–109.
8. Ibid.
9. Gordon, J. S., Staples, J. K., Blyta, A., Bytyqi, M., and Wilson, A. T., "Treatment of Posttraumatic Stress Disorder in Postwar Kosovar Adolescents Using Mind-Body Skills Groups: A Randomized Controlled Trial," *Journal of Clinical Psychiatry* 69, no. 9 (2008): 1469–1476.
10. Gerbarg, Wallace, and Brown, "Mass Disasters."

Chapter 5

1. Peng, Robert, *Qigong Master: My Life and Secret Teachings* (New York: Rainbow Tree Publishing, 2010).
2. Craig, A. D., "How Do You Feel—Now? The Anterior Insula and Human Awareness," *Nature Reviews Neuroscience* 10, no. 1 (2009): 59–70; Craig, A. D., "Interoception and Emotion," in *Handbook of Emotions*, 3rd ed., edited by M. Lewis, J. M. Haviland-Jones, and L. F. Barrett (New

York: Guilford, 2008), 272–288; Craig, A. D., "Interoception: The Sense of the Physiological Condition of the Body," *Current Opinion in Neurobiology* 13, no. 4 (2003): 500–505; Critchley, H. D., "Neural Mechanisms of Autonomic, Affective, and Cognitive Integration," *Journal of Comparative Neurology* 93, no. 1 (2005): 154–166.

Chapter 6

1. Carter, C. S., "Neuroendocrine Perspectives on Social Attachment and Love," *Psychoneuroendocrinology* 23, no. 8 (1998): 779–818; Carter, C. S., Grippo, A. J., Pournajafi-Nazarloo, H., Ruscio, M. G., and Porges, S. W., "Oxytocin, Vasopressin, and Sociability," *Progress in Brain Research* 170 (2008): 331–336; Porges, S. W., "The Polyvagal Theory: Phylogenetic Substrates of a Social Nervous System," *International Journal of Psychophysiology* 42, no. 2 (2001): 123–146.
2. Bucci, W., "Pathways of Emotional Communication," *Psychoanalytic Inquiry* 20 (2001): 40–70.
3. Carter, S., "Neuroendocrine Perspectives."
4. Fehmi, L. G., and McKnight, J. T., "Attention and Neurofeedback Synchrony Training: Clinical Results and Their Significance," *Journal of Neurotherapy* 5, no. 1–2 (2001): 45–62.
5. Hummel, F., and Gerloff, C., "Larger Interregional Synchrony Is Associated with Greater Behavioral Success in a Complex Sensory Integration Task in Humans," *Cerebral Cortex* 15, no. 5 (2005): 670–678.
6. Espinoza, Cholene, *Through the Eye of the Storm* (White River Juction, VT: Chelsea Green, 2006), and from e-mail correspondence.
7. Brown, R. P., and Gerbarg, P. L., "Sudarshan Kriya Yogic Breathing, Part 1"; "Sudarshan Kriya Yogic Breathing in the Treatment of Stress, Anxiety, and Depression: Part 2 — Clinical Applications and Guidelines," *Journal of Alternative and Complementary Medicine* 11, no. 4 (2005): 711–717.
8. Craig, "How Do You Feel — Now?"; Craig, "Interoception and Emotion"; Craig, "Interoception: The Sense of the Physiological Condition of the Body."
9. Streeter, C. C., Whitfield, T. H., Owen, L., Rein, T., Karri, S. K., Yakhkind, A., Perlmutter, R., Prescot, A., Renshaw, P. F., Ciraulo, D. A., and Jensen, J. E., "Effects of Yoga versus Walking on Mood, Anxiety, and Brain GABA Levels: A Randomized Controlled MRS Study," *Journal of Alternative and Complementary Medicine* 16, no. 11 (2010): 1145–1152.

Chapter 7

1. Peters, C., Spahn, C., and Aschendorff, A., "Music Performance Anxiety. A Review of the Literature," inaugural dissertation of the Faculty of Medicine presented at the University of Freiburg, Germany, 2009, www.freidok.uni-freiburg.de/volltexte/6603/pdf/MPA.pdf.
2. Bernardi, L., Schneider, A., Pomidori, L., Paolucci, E., and Cogo, A., "Hypoxic Ventilatory Response in Successful Extreme Altitude Climbers," *European Respiratory Journal* 27, no. 1 (2006): 165–171.
3. Peng, Robert, *Qigong Master: My Life and Secret Teachings* (New York: Rainbow Tree Publishing, 2010).

References

Beauchaine, T. P. "Vagal Tone, Development, and Gray's Motivational Theory: Toward an Integrated Model of Autonomic Nervous System Functioning in Psychopathology." *Developmental Psychopathology* 13, no. 2 (2001): 183–214.

Beauchaine, T. P., Katkin, E. S., Strassberg, Z., and Snarr, J. "Disinhibitory Psychopathology in Male Adolescents: Discriminating Conduct Disorder from Attention-Deficit/Hyperactivity Disorder through Concurrent Assessment of Multiple Autonomic States." *Journal of Abnormal Psychology* 110, no. 4 (2001): 610–624.

Benson, T. (1996). *Timeless Healing: The Power and Biology of Belief,* 222–234. New York: Scribners, 1996.

Bernardi, L., Gabutti, A., Porta, C., and Spicuzza, L. "Slow Breathing Reduces Chemoreflex Response to Hypoxia and Hypercapnia, and Increases Baroreflex Sensitivity." *Journal of Hypertension* 19, no. 12 (2001): 2221–2229.

Bernardi, L., Schneider, A., Pomidori, L., Paolucci, E., and Cogo, A. "Hypoxic Ventilatory Response in Successful Extreme Altitude Climbers." *European Respiratory Journal* 27, no. 1 (2006): 165–171.

Bernardi, L., Sleight, P., Bandinelli, G., Cencetti, S., Fattorini, L., Wdowczyc-Szulc, J., and Lagi, A. "Effect of Rosary Prayer and Yoga Mantras on Autonomic Cardiovascular Rhythms: A Comparative Study." Health Module, *British Medical Journal* 323, no. 7327 (2001): 1446.

Berntson, G. G., Sarter, M., and Cacioppo, J. T. "Ascending Visceral Regulation of Cortical Affective Information Processing." *European Journal Neuroscience* 18, no. 8 (2003): 2103–2109.

Brianchaninov, I. *On the Prayer of Jesus*. Translated by Father Lazarus. Boston, MA: New Seeds, 2006.

Brown, R. P., and Gerbarg, P. L. *Non-Drug Treatments for ADHD: Options for Kids, Adults, and Clinicians*. W. W. Norton: New York, in press.

———. "Sudarshan Kriya Yogic Breathing in the Treatment of Stress, Anxiety, and Depression: Part 1 — Neurophysiologic Model." *Journal of Alternative and Complementary Medicine* 11, no. 1 (2005): 189–201.

———. "Sudarshan Kriya Yogic Breathing in the Treatment of Stress, Anxiety, and Depression: Part 2 — Clinical Applications and Guidelines." *Journal of Alternative and Complementary Medicine* 11, no. 4 (2005): 711–717.

———. "Yoga Breathing, Meditation, and Longevity." In *Longevity, Regeneration, and Optimal Health* (Annals of the New York Academy of Sciences, vol. 1172), edited by C. Bushell, E. L. Olivo, and N. D. Theise. Boston, MA: Wiley-Blackwell, 2009.

Brown, R. P., Gerbarg, P. L., and Muskin, Philip R. *How to Use Herbs, Nutrients, and Yoga in Mental Health Care*. W. W. Norton: New York, 2009.

Brown, R. P., Gerbarg, P. L., Vermani, M., and Katzman, M. "First Trial of Breathing, Movement, and Meditation for PTSD, Depression, and Anxiety Related to September 11th New York City World Trade Center Attacks." Lecture given at the annual meeting of the American Psychiatric Association, New Orleans, LA, May 22, 2010.

Brown, R. P., Gerbarg, P. L., Vermani, M., and Katzman, M. "Second Trial of Breathing, Movement, and Meditation PTSD, Depression, and Anxiety Related to September 11th New York City World Trade Center Attacks." Lecture given at the annual meeting of the American Psychiatric Association, New Orleans, LA, May 22, 2010.

Bucci, W. "Pathways of Emotional Communication." *Psychoanalytic Inquiry* 20 (2001): 40–70.

Calabrese, P., Perrault, H., Dinh, T. P., Eberhard, A., and Benchetrit, G. "Cardio-respiratory Interactions during Resistive Load Breathing." *American Journal of Physiology: Regulatory, Integrative and Comparative Physiology* 279, no. 6 (2000): R2208–R2213.

Cappo, B. M., and Holmes, D. S. "The Utility of Prolonged Respiratory Exhalation for Reducing Physiological and Psychological Arousal in Nonthreatening and Threatening Situations." *Journal of Psychosomatic Research* 28, no. 4 (1984): 265–273.

Carter, C. S. "Neuroendocrine Perspectives on Social Attachment and Love." *Psychoneuroendocrinology* 23, no. 8 (1998): 779–818.

Carter, C. S., Grippo, A. J., Pournajafi-Nazarloo, H., Ruscio, M. G., and Porges, S. W. "Oxytocin, Vasopressin, and Sociability." *Progress in Brain Research* 170 (2008): 331–336.

Clark, M. E., and Hirschman, R. "Effects of Paced Respiration on Anxiety Reduction in a Clinical Population." *Biofeedback Self-Regulation* 15, no. 3 (1990): 273–284.

Craig, A. D. "How Do You Feel—Now? The Anterior Insula and Human Awareness." *Nature Reviews Neuroscience* 10, no. 1 (2009): 59–70.

Craig, A. D. "Interoception and Emotion." In *Handbook of Emotions*, 3rd ed., edited by M. Lewis, J. M. Haviland-Jones, and L. F. Barrett, 272–288. New York: Guilford, 2008.

Craig, A. D. "Interoception: The Sense of the Physiological Condition of the Body." *Current Opinion in Neurobiology* 13, no. 4 (2003): 500–505.

Critchley, H. D. "Neural Mechanisms of Autonomic, Affective, and Cognitive Integration." *Journal of Comparative Neurology* 93, no. 1 (2005): 154–166.

Damasio, R. R. *The Feeling of What Happens: Body and Emotion in the Making of Consciousness.* New York: Harcourt Brace, 1999.

Das, P., Kemp, A. H., Liddell, B. J., Olivieri, G., Peduto, A., Gordon, E., and Williams, L. M. "Pathways for Fear Perception: Modulation of Amygdala Activity by Thalamo-Cortical Systems." *NeuroImage* 26 (2005): 141–148.

Descilo, T., Vedamurtachar, A., Gerbarg, P. L., Nagaraja, D., Gangadhar, B. N. G., Damodaran, B., Adelson, B., Braslow, L. H., Marcus, M., and Brown, R. P. "Effects of a Yoga-Breath Intervention Alone and in Combination with an Exposure Therapy for PTSD and Depression in Survivors of the 2004 Southeast Asia Tsunami." *Acta Psychiatrica Scandinavica* 121, no. 4 (2010): 289–300.

Elliot, S., and Edmonson, D. *Coherent Breathing: The Definitive Method, Theory, and Practice.* Allen, TX: Coherence Press, 2008.

Espinoza, Cholene. *Through the Eye of the Storm.* White River Junction, VT: Chelsea Green, 2006.

Fehmi, L. G., and McKnight, J. T. "Attention and Neurofeedback Synchrony Training: Clinical Results and Their Significance." *Journal of Neurotherapy* 5, no. 1–2 (2001): 45–62.

Fehmi, Les, and Robbins, Jim. *Dissolving Pain: Simple Brain-Training Exercises for Overcoming Chronic Pain.* Boston, MA: Trumpeter Books, 2010.

Fehmi, Les, and Robbins, Jim. *The Open-Focus Brain.* Boston, MA: Trumpeter Books, 2007.

Gerbarg, P. L. "Yoga and Neuro-Psychoanalysis." In *Bodies in Treatment: The*

Unspoken Dimension, edited by F. S. Anderson, 132–133. Hillsdale, NJ: Analytic Press, 2007.

Gerbarg, P. L., and Brown, R. P. "Yoga: A Breath of Relief for Hurricane Katrina Refugees." *Current Psychiatry* 4, no. 10 (2005): 55–67.

Gerbarg, P. L., Wallace, G. S., and Brown, R. P. "Mass Disasters and Mind-Body Solutions: Evidence and Field Insights." *International Journal of Yoga Therapy* 21 (2011): 97–109.

Gordon, J. S., Staples, J. K., Blyta, A., Bytyqi, M., and Wilson, A. T. "Treatment of Posttraumatic Stress Disorder in Postwar Kosovar Adolescents Using Mind-Body Skills Groups: A Randomized Controlled Trial." *Journal of Clinical Psychiatry* 69, no. 9 (2008): 1469–1476.

Hassett, A. L., Radvanski, D. C., Vaschillo, E. G., Vaschillo, B., Sigal, L. H., Karavidas, M. K., Buyske, S., and Lehrer, P. M. "A Pilot Study of the Efficacy of Heart Rate Variability (HRV) Biofeedback in Patients with Fibromyalgia." *Applied Psychophysiology Biofeedback* 32, no. 1 (2007): 1–10.

Hummel, F., and Gerloff, C. "Larger Interregional Synchrony Is Associated with Greater Behavioral Success in a Complex Sensory Integration Task in Humans." *Cerebral Cortex* 15, no. 5 (2005): 670–678.

Kalyani, B. G, Venkatasubramanian, G., Arasappa, R., Rao, N. P., Kalmady, S. V., Behere, R. V., Rao, H., Vasudev, M. K., and Gangadhar, B. N. "Neurohemodynamic Correlates of 'OM' Chanting: A Pilot Functional Magnetic Resonance Imaging Study." *International Journal of Yoga* 4, no. 1 (2011): 3–6.

Kuntsevich, V., Bushell, W. C., and Theise, N. D. "Mechanisms of Yogic Practices in Health, Aging, and Disease." *Mount Sinai Journal of Medicine* 77, no. 5 (2010): 559–569.

Larsen, S., Yee, W., Gerbarg, P. L., Brown, R. P., Gunkelman, J., and Sherlin, L. Unpublished paper presented at the annual meeting of the American Psychiatric Association, Toronto, Canada (May 20–25, 2006).

Lehrer, P., Sasaki, Y., and Saito, Y. "Zazen and Cardiac Variability." *Psychosomatic Medicine* 61, no. 6 (1999): 812–821.

Peng, Robert. *Qigong Master: My Life and Secret Teachings.* New York. Rainbow Tree, 2010.

Peng, Robert. *Four Golden Wheels.* Audio DVD. www.robertpeng.com.

Peters, C., Spahn, C., and Aschendorff, A. "Music Performance Anxiety. A Review of the Literature." Inaugural dissertation of the Faculty of Medicine presented at the University of Freiburg, Germany, 2009. www.freidok.uni-freiburg.de/volltexte/6603/pdf/MPA.pdf.

Philippot, P., Gaetane, C., and Blairy, S. "Respiratory Feedback in the Generation of Emotion." *Cognition and Emotion* 16, no. 5 (2002): 605–607.

Porges, S. W. "The Polyvagal Theory: New Insights into Adaptive Reactions of the Autonomic Nervous System." *Cleveland Clinic Journal of Medicine* 76, no. 2 (2009): S86–S90.

Porges, S. W. "The Polyvagal Theory: Phylogenetic Substrates of a Social Nervous System." *International Journal of Psychophysiology* 42, no. 2 (2001): 123–146.

Streeter, C. C., Whitfield, T. H., Owen, L., Rein, T., Karri, S. K., Yakhkind, A., Perlmutter, R., Prescot, A., Renshaw, P. F., Ciraulo, D. A., and Jensen, J. E. "Effects of Yoga versus Walking on Mood, Anxiety, and Brain GABA Levels: A Randomized Controlled MRS Study." *Journal of Alternative and Complementary Medicine* 16, no. 11 (2010): 1145–1152.

Streeter, C. C., Gerbarg, P. L., and Brown, R. P. "Mind-Body Training for Health Care Providers in Areas of Mississippi Affected by the 2010 Gulf Oil Spill." Poster presentation given at the Symposium on Yoga Research, Stockbridge, MA, September 23–25, 2011.

Telles, S., Singh, N., Joshi, M., and Balkrishna, A. "Posttraumatic Stress Symptoms and Heart Rate Variability in Bihar Flood Survivors following Yoga: A Randomized Controlled Study." *BioMed Central Psychiatry* 10, no. 1 (2010). Retrieved from www.biomedcentral.com/1471-244X/10/18.

Thayer, J. F., and Brosschot, J. F. "Psychosomatics and Psychopathology: Looking Up and Down from the Brain." *Psychoneuroendocrinology* 30, no. 10 (2005): 1050–1058.

Vasiliev, Vladimir. *Let Every Breath . . . Secrets of the Russian Breath Masters.* Richmond Hill, Ontario: Russian Martial Art, 2006.

Weintraub, A. *Yoga for Depression.* New York: Broadway Books Random House, 2004.

Yu, J. "Airway Mechanosensors." *Respiratory Physiology Neurobiology* 148, no. 3 (2005): 217–243.

Index

The letter *t* following a page number denotes a table.

in Sudan, 79–80
used as an anchor, 18
ways to use, 17–18
See also Total Breath; specific topics
community resiliency, building, 84
computer use, 53–54
connection and disconnection, 113–16
Craig, Bud, 119, 120

daily activity, Coherent Breathing during, 17–18
Deepwater Horizon oil spill, 73–74
Deng, Luka, 79, 80
disease, 85–86

Elliot, Stephen, 16, 26
Espinoza, Cholene, 113–16

families breathing together, 25–26
family needs and breathing practice, 22
fear. See anxiety
Fehmi, Les, 105, 112
Feldenkrais, 126
first responders, 55–56
flood in Bihar, India, 72
"freeze" reaction, 117

GABA (gamma-aminobutyric acid), 120–21
Gandhi, Mahatma, 2
generalized anxiety disorder (GAD), 65–66
Gerbarg, Patricia L., 22, 25, 61–62, 117–18, 130
fear of public speaking, 64–65
Global Grassroots' Academy for Conscious Change in Rwanda, 78
golf, 129–30

Gordon, James, 81–82
ground-glass lungs, 71
Ground Zero workers, 56
Gulf of Mexico oil spill, 73–74

"Ha" Breath, 91, 135–36
ADHD and, 89–90
awakening your system with, 88–89
case material, 76–77, 90
how and when to use, 89, 146t
order of practice and, 149–52t
"Ha" breathing, contraindications to, 89
Haiti earthquake of 2010, 74–77
head rolls, Resistance Breathing with, 50–51
Healing Power of the Breath CD, 6, 15–16, 39, 44, 56, 63
heart rate variability (HRV), Coherent Breathing and, 10–12
high-altitude performance, 128–29
hypercapnia, 127–28
hypoxia, 127–28

illness, 85–86
Indian Ocean tsunami of 2004, 72–73
insomnia, Coherent Breathing for, 17
intimacy, 42

Jesus Prayer, 2, 44
Johnson, Barbara, 76–77, 81

Katzman, Martin, 66, 70–71

Lao Tzu, 9
Larsen, Stephen, 112
Lee, Bruce, 2
lung disease, 5

getting closer with, 42
with head rolls, 50–51
how and when to use, 143t, 145t,
    148t
hurting the throat, 41
obstacles to, 40–42
and peak artistic performance, 127
with shoulder rolls, 51
and sleep, 47
trying too hard, 41–42
See also Total Breath
Respire-1 CD, 7, 16, 61, 81, 90, 129
Rwanda, Coherent Breathing in, 77–78

September 11 World Trade Center
    attacks, 69–71, 113, 114
Serving Those Who Serve (STWS),
    55–56, 69
sexual trauma, 116–20
shoulder rolls, Resistance Breathing
    with, 51
sleep, Resistance Breathing and, 47
sleep apnea, 24
sleep time, breathing for, 61
sleeping, thinking instead of, 62
sleeping difficulty, Coherent Breathing
    for, 17
Slow Down CD, 7, 15–16, 26, 27
slowing down, instructions for, 27–28
song, kong, tong, dong, 101–4, 136, 147t
sports injuries, 56
Stackman, Marshall Saul, 69
S.T.A.R.T. Clinic for Mood and Anxi-
    ety Disorders, 65–66
Streeter, Chris, 74, 121
stress
    caregiver, 81

negative emotions and, 59–61
    See also post-traumatic stress
        disorder
stressful relationships, 108–10
stretching, 50, 52–54, 92, 148t
Sudan, Coherent Breathing in, 79–80
Sudarshan Kriya Yoga (SKY), 66
sustainability, 81–83

Telles, Shirley, 72
Total Breath, 4–5, 48–50, 56–57, 133–34
    case material, 63
    how and when to use, 85, 145t
    om and, 101
    and stress, 59, 85
transformation using Western scien
    tific paradigms, 111–12
trauma
    how breathing may resolve, 119–21
    inoculating against the effects of,
        83–85
    See also mass disasters; post-trau-
        matic stress disorder
tsunami in Southeast Asia (2004),
    72–73

ujjayi. *See* Resistance Breathing

Vasiliev, Vladimir, 44
Vermani, Monica, 66, 70–71
Vibration Breathing, 136
    how and when to use, 147
    See also *om*; *song, kong, tong, dong*
vibrations
    breathing with good, 97–98
    moving them to different parts of
        body, 104–5